Praise for Kate McLaughlin

Profound and poetically written, this book takes the reader on a journey that begins in the home of a happy and loving family, and devolves dramatically as first one, and than the other teenage child onsets with severe symptoms of bipolar disorder.

Kate McLaughlin, telling her story through her diary and keen sensibility, uncannily captures both the words and internal feelings of her children. For the first time, a reader sees not only the impact of a child's illness on a family, but also the impact of one sibling's illness on the other.

Yet, in the fullness of time, the family learns to navigate the illness, the children become well, and this beautiful memoir offers hope and encouragement to every parent and adolescent who is forced to take this reluctant journey. We highly recommend this book.

~Demitri F. Papolos, M.D. and Janice Papolos, co-authors of *The Bipolar Child*

Lovingly dedicated to the kids,
Anna, and Rick

With thanks to
Barbro, Gina, Margi, the Papolos', and Sally

To Ann Whitcher-Gentzke—
With Appreciation for your work
that ultimately benefits my
loved ones.

Kate McLaughlin

This is a story of hope.
A story of love and determination,
it is a story of found peace.

"The most beautiful people we have known are those who have known defeat, known suffering, known struggle, known loss, and have found their way out of the depths. These people have an appreciation, sensitivity, and an understanding of life that fills them with compassion, gentleness, and a deep, loving concern. Beautiful people do not just happen."

— Elisabeth Kuebler Ross

Prologue

I began writing this book to heal myself and clarify my observations and memories about raising children with mental illness. I soon realized that, despite the serious topic and the gravity of our trials, telling this story could help the estimated 1.9 million Americans age fifteen and over living with Bipolar Disorder. In addition to mental illness, hundreds of thousands of families deal with debilitating physical illness, emotional disorders, and teenage rebellion. Most endure great challenges, often feeling isolated and alone. It is my hope that those parents and family members who read our story will be encouraged, and that those who have suffered or are suffering regain a sense of joy and purpose.

As our family blindly wended our way down an unfamiliar, sometimes harrowing route, we would have benefited, perhaps felt less frightened, had someone before us shared their notes from a similar journey traveled. By writing about our experiences and sharing our progress, I aim to reassure and encourage you and, ultimately, alleviate some of the fear that naturally accompanies the challenges of living with Bipolar Disorder.

This desire heightened as I read other books written by parents whose children were chronically ill. When I finished one of these accounts feeling sad and disappointed, I realized that I saw the experience so differently. It is hard to live with mental illness, with any illness. I know the implicit challenges. However, I also know the rich blessings we receive by living graciously and lovingly with anything, everything. I know the potential for peace and contentment. We hear too little about what is possible in the midst of chronic illness, particularly mental illness, and it is this good news that I share.

Do I wish my children were healthy, free from mental illness? Yes, of course. Would I change it if I had the necessary magical incantation? Tough call. Are their lives, our life, less glorious because they have Bipolar Disorder? Not one bit. In fact, it may be more glorious because they do. I don't know. But I do know that, thanks in part to medical advances, we enjoy innumerable good times, deep and abiding love, and a greater respect for diversity and individuality that many of our contemporaries have yet to discover. I know that every difficulty has nurtured strength, or character, or both. We have a keen appreciation of one another and of simply being together.

I sometimes think my children are highly evolved spirits who came to exist before this world was prepared for them. They are sensitive. They know more than people do twice their age. They tune into feelings and emotions on a higher frequency than others. They are, in many ways, advanced. Would I take that away for them to be "average?" Would you?

Rather than ponder impossibilities and dwell on "what ifs," I revel in the wonder. I live in love and in the light. I invite you to travel these pages with us and share in our evolution, so that you, too, can learn some of the important lessons we have learned along the way.

Good tidings.
-KL McLaughlin

1
Before

"I accept life unconditionally. Life holds so much — so much to be so happy about always. Most people ask for happiness on condition. Happiness can be felt only if you do not set conditions."
— Arthur Rubenstein

We had so much to be happy about. Our life, before Bipolar Disorder's rude intrusion, was nearly ideal. My husband Mark and I had been a couple since high school. After dating through college, we married at the time I got my first teaching job. Mark finished his degree a few months later and soon began climbing the corporate ladder. Eager to make a life for ourselves, Mark worked long hours while I taught school and took graduate classes. In just a couple of years, we had our first child and our first home. Although we felt grown up and responsible, we were naïve and young. We excitedly approached parenting assuming we would spend the next twenty-plus years shaping our children into contributing adults. Despite family trees heavily weighted with serious mental illness, alcoholism, and substance abuse, we thought we would avoid these difficult and stigmatizing issues.

My first pregnancy was uneventful, and our seven-pound, four-ounce Chloe was born with a perfectly shaped head crowned with downy, blonde hair. She had big blue eyes above a button nose, and a pink rosebud mouth.

Chloe drew admiration from the gallery outside the hospital nursery. One man, a father gazing over from his own newborn, smiled and said, "She is the most beautiful baby I've ever seen. She's even prettier than mine."

Chloe was as difficult as she was pretty. She reacted to every change in her environment, whether it was fluorescent lighting when we stepped into a shop or the wind on her skin as we walked outdoors.

One day, with a lengthy shopping list and four-month-old Chloe, I headed out. As if on cue, she began crying when the sun hit her face, settling down as we got to the car. Once confined to her car seat, she cried some more. The drive to the supermarket soothed her, but the process of getting out of the car and into a cart got her going again. She calmed down, but as soon as we passed through the front doors, she wailed. On the first aisle, an older woman approached us, looked at Chloe's pinched, tear-streaked face, and said, "Oh, sweet thing, I hate to hear you cry, but you're so pretty, it just doesn't matter."

Aisle after aisle I alternately carried Chloe in my arms and jostled her in her infant seat. She continued to cry. As we neared the end of our list, we passed the same woman who looked at me, looked at Chloe, and then said, "Honey, nobody's that pretty."

Chloe's fussiness baffled my mom and grandmother, each of whom had four children. She cried dozens of times a day. If it got hotter, colder, brighter, darker, noisier, or breezier, Chloe cried. She never slept more than three hours at a time, wanted to eat more often than that, and only napped for an hour or two each day. This continued until she crawled at six months. Finally, with some independent mobility, she cried less often.

Chloe's happiness increased rapidly as she grasped language and began communicating in earnest. She developed a large vocabulary by age one and spoke complete sentences at eighteen months, but she did not sleep through the night until she was three. Despite her difficult infancy, Chloe was a joy, adding a new dimension to our lives. Mark and I adored her. I went back to teaching when the new school year began and she stayed with a babysitter who loved her, too. We chattered on the way to and from work, and she knew all the street names en route before she was two. We often stopped for a drink or a snack, and sometimes a jaunt in the park. I loved being in her company, delighted by her rapidly expanding intellect and warm, loving personality.

On weekends, Chloe joined Mark and me as we worked on the house and in the yard, turning our fixer-upper into a prize. She liked going to Home Depot and the lumberyard, and loved to see her grandparents on Sundays. She noticed everything around her, asked questions, and learned at an unbelievable rate. Mark and I were devoted and amazed. She was the center of our world. In fact, I remember worrying that I might not be able to love another child as much as I loved her. However, that was not the case.

Two weeks past Chloe's third birthday, Michael arrived. Born two weeks late, and after only three hours of labor, this musty-yet-sweet-smelling, blue-eyed, blond-haired person immediately stole my heart. When I first held him in my arms, I felt doubly blessed. We had a daughter and a son. Perfect.

Despite frequent respiratory ailments and difficulty keeping meals down, Michael was an easy baby. He ate regularly and slept through the night at six weeks. He took long naps during the day and, when awake, smiled more often than not. Most things fascinated and amused him. Changes that drove his sister into a crying frenzy at that age did not faze him. An easy-going child, he loved sitting in my arms as much as he liked lying on a blanket with his toys.

Michael adored Chloe and she marveled at him. Reveling in her role as big sister, she held him and talked to him as often as she could. Early mornings and after naps, Chloe climbed into Michael's crib, smoothed his hair, tickled his chin, read to him, and talked to him. She was precociously responsible and he trusted her. They quickly grew into playmates.

Two weeks after Michael turned three we welcomed another blessing into our family. Monica entered the world kicking and screaming, and continued to do so for the next twenty-four hours. Once she settled down, she was the easiest baby I had ever encountered. Six-year-old Chloe and three-year-old Michael were prepared and excited. Throughout the pregnancy we read books and had dozens of conversations about babies. We toured the hospital maternity ward and newborn nursery, and the staff talked to the children about the day our baby would arrive. When she did, our family felt complete.

Monica loved it when we held her and we loved holding her. She ate well, slept well, and smiled early and often. Chloe and Michael fawned over their baby sister. They talked to her, tried to make her laugh, anticipated her needs, and encouraged her as she learned new skills. A kindergartener, Chloe wanted to bring Monica to class for share time. Michael was thrilled to stay home with Monica and me, rather than go to the babysitter. When Chloe returned from school, she and Michael played with Monica before Chloe headed off to do her own thing and Michael spent time with neighborhood friends. The three of them bonded instantly and intensely.

Wanting to spend my days with our three children, I left my public-school career behind and ran a part-time preschool at home. We spent our days learning and exploring, going to parks and wilderness areas, taking long walks, reading dozens of books, and constantly talking. All three children developed extensive vocabularies and read early.

We grew vegetable and flower gardens, cooked and baked, had preschool at home three mornings a week, and loved each other a lot. By the time Mark got home from work I was tired, so he played with the children and helped clear up after dinner. Together we read bedtime stories, got the kids tucked in, and enjoyed long, quiet evenings at home. We frequently marveled at our good luck.

As the children grew and the demands of Mark's career increased, we strove to find balance between work and play. Mark coached Michael's Little League teams and I helped in classrooms. We took family vacations every year, often traveling to spend holidays with aunts, uncles, and cousins. No matter what challenges we faced, including a job transfer that moved us hundreds of miles from family and friends, we managed to maintain an even keel. If you encountered us in the mall, you would have seen a happy, upper-middle-class family enjoying the American dream. We had it all.

Once all three children were in school I volunteered in the community as well as their classrooms. To pursue my own interests, I took the Master Gardening course at the local university, and then volunteered to share what I had learned with the public. I wrote every day, although mostly for myself, and read voraciously. Then I received my first book deal and began working on that. All the while, Mark continued to advance in his career, assuming more responsibility and loving every minute of it.

Chloe, Michael, and Monica were great kids, and still are exceptional people. They each worked hard in school, earning good grades and praise from their teachers. They played sports, got along well with others, and were, for the most part, obedient. They helped around the house, did the chores listed on their charts without much prodding, and cooperated well. I was grateful for this. Discord and hostility had marred my own childhood, and I wanted this phase of my life to be different. We really did have a happy family. Our lives seemed charmed. We never encountered anything that we couldn't figure out together — that is, until we encountered chronic mental illness.

Until we encountered insanity.

2
Spring 1999

"... mighty things from small beginnings grow."
—John Dryden

As is often the case with mental illness, the beginning is difficult to pinpoint. When Mark and I got married and decided to have children, our goals and aspirations were simple. We wanted a loving, kind, intelligent relationship with one another, and mutually respectful and appreciative relationships with our children. More than anything, we wanted to be happy. We never discussed, never even considered, obstacles that might be beyond our control. A naïve optimism and youthful sense of empowerment encouraged us to overlook the ramifications of our parent's ills and choices.

Even though depression was common in my family, my father and one brother were alcoholic and drug addicted, and Mark's mom had a chronic mental illness that we did not understand, it never occurred to us that those diseases would re-emerge in our children. We assumed that choice and circumstance played major roles in our childhood families' problems. With my child-development and education background, and Mark's capable self-assurance, we confidently thought that expert nurture would overcome any detriments of nature. The now obvious possibilities never crossed our minds.

In hindsight, scores of indicators and a condemning genetic history practically screamed warnings of ultimate mental illness in our children. But we did not know something was wrong until Bipolar Disorder roared into our lives, beginning its insidious march through what we thought was right and good and forcing us to reexamine our ideas about family, success, spirituality ... and even love.

Seventeen-year-old Chloe was an exuberant five-foot, two-inch, blue-eyed brunette entering her junior year in high school, sights set on maintaining academic excellence and going to college at NYU or USC. An exceptional student with a quick mind and an uncanny understanding of complex issues, she earned a 3.86 GPA while taking honors and advanced placement classes, playing and coaching soccer, and serving as a yearbook editor. I smile when I recall a parent-teacher conference during which her calculus, English, and journalism teachers each assured me that she excelled in their specific subject and would excel there in college and the work world.

Everyone envisioned Chloe achieving exceptional goals and making significant contributions. People expected her to change the world. She was articulate, well read, curious, and doggedly determined. These traits served her well as she pursued her intellectual goals. She had an amazing mind.

In the spring of 1999, Chloe added a part-time job at a local resort to her already busy schedule. With a reputation for exceptional service and client care, the resort offered a safe place for students to work at far above minimum wage. The schedule was good because she arrived early on weekends and worked the morning shift, or started in the afternoon and worked until only nine or ten. It was coming home from work one night that she had her first car accident, likely symptomatic of her first severe manic phase.

Turning left at an intersection, Chloe broadsided a Volvo coming from the opposite direction. At the time, in shock and filled with anxiety, she claimed not to have seen the car. Had she not seen it, or had she thought she could beat it through the intersection, misjudging its rate of speed and her ability to turn and accelerate? Several months later, even she examined these possibilities. At any rate, the accident was significant enough to total the Volvo and seriously damage our truck. Luckily, both Chloe and the other driver escaped injury.

Within days of that accident, she had another mishap, sideswiping a street sign, while distracted by a car for sale on the side of the road. Was this typical teenage behavior? Since she was our eldest, Mark and I thought it might be, but I had a nagging suspicion that something was not right. Although often clumsy, Chloe had never before been careless or unfocused. From infancy, Chloe was hyper-aware of her surroundings, and could recall and recount details with uncanny accuracy. I will never forget one of many conversations I had with her pediatrician before she began to crawl.

"Dr. Gillian, I'm so frustrated. I feel like I'm doing something wrong. Chloe cries all the time. I can settle her down pretty quickly, but then something else sets her off and she's crying again."

Patiently, and with sincere interest, Dr. Gillian asked, "What do you mean when you say something sets her off?"

"For the longest time I couldn't pinpoint it, because it varied so much. Then I realized it was change, change to anything, everything. She fusses with sudden changes in light, whether brighter or darker. If we leave a building and it's hot out, she cries. If we enter a room that's too cool, the same thing happens. When I undress her to change her diaper or bathe her, she cries. I know the minute she wets her diaper, because she shivers and starts crying. She's more sensitive to the world around her than I ever thought a baby would be."

Dr. Gillian's eyes sparkled in a grandmotherly way as she enthusiastically explained, "You are so lucky. Chloe is exceptionally bright. She observes and understands her surroundings and becomes overwhelmed by the sensory input. Her still undeveloped nervous system can't process everything, so she cries. Don't worry so much about her well-being or your mothering skills. As she gets older, this will improve. Be happy and excited that you have such an intelligent child. Learn to ease Chloe into new situations and the two of you will be just fine."

Grateful for the kind, insightful pep talk, I relaxed and tried to follow Dr. Gillian's advice, which proved to be right on the money. In the intervening years, Chloe's responses to new stimuli toned down. By the time she started kindergarten, she handled disruptions and distractions with few problems. Until now.

Along with the car accidents, a new level of moodiness settled in and Chloe grew increasingly clumsy and forgetful. She tripped on, dropped, knocked over, and lost things at a comical pace. I began to worry, questioning behaviors and choices that I would previously have overlooked. Then my worries seemed unfounded as my girl, although inordinately distracted and excessively on the go, finished her junior year with accolades and no more problems on the road or elsewhere.

With no summer classes and extra time on her hands, Chloe picked up additional shifts at work. Her social life picked up, too, since a group of workmates developed a routine of going out after work, drinking coffee, watching movies, or just hanging out. Her routine grew more hectic, her calendar more full. The hours with friends and movie watching increased, allowing only a few hours of sleep before she was back out the door to work or to play. Even though they represented a change in her routine, at the time Chloe's activities seemed within a normal range for a young woman her age.

The only problem that continually vexed us was Chloe's sudden use of foul language. Not being a family that curses with abandon, we were shocked when she regularly accessorized comments and conversations with four-letter words. Aside from that, there did not seem to be anything wrong. Mark and I were confident that Chloe was not drinking or doing drugs. We often talked to the children about expectations, and Chloe was open and honest, making good choices, and honoring commitments.

Despite her busy schedule and lack of sleep, she remained upbeat and energetic. Before now, she had always required eight to ten hours a night. Now she got five or six. Nevertheless, she kept going with a smile on her face, working most days, going out until midnight every night, watching movies when she returned, sleeping a few hours, and then starting all over again. Sometimes she stayed awake all night and seemed unaffected by wear. When we talked about her new routines, Chloe glowed with enthusiasm and excitement. She seemed thrilled with her life and intent on enjoying every minute of it. I didn't realize we were on the threshold of radical change.

3
Summer 1999

"Discomfort guides my tongue
And bids me speak of nothing but despair."
— William Shakespeare

In a few short weeks, Chloe's demeanor changed. Suddenly argumentative and contentious at home, she grew angry and inconsiderate of others. She bickered with fourteen-year-old Michael and eleven-year-old Monica over insignificant things, taking their comments personally and negatively. Mornings, her music blared, even though the other children agreed to get up later so she had full use of the bathroom. When confronted about her thoughtlessness, she replied confidently, "So what, Mom. They can get up. Tell them to eat breakfast or something. If it's not too early for me, it's not too early for them. But they can't use the bathroom until I'm done."

Most afternoons brought conflict. Chloe flew into the house after school, tossed her backpack on the floor, and headed for the TV remote. It did not matter who was watching what. She picked up the remote and changed the channel.

"Hey, I was watching that," Michael shot out one day. "You can't just come in and change the channel."

"I just did. I've been working hard at school and this is the only time I have to relax and watch TV, so you'll just have to live with it."

"We went to school, too, and we want to watch our show. You have to wait your turn."

With an air of bravado making it clear that her wants took precedence over theirs, she retorted, "This *is* my turn you stupid little brat."

Chloe had outgrown name-calling years ago, but it suddenly returned to common practice, and I resented dealing with immature behaviors from a child who had always seemed older than her years. Chloe became difficult to talk with, sometimes tough to be around. She stomped rather than walked and treated every expression of interest as an invasion of privacy or a criticism. She was often grandiose.

"How did you do on your English essay today?" I once asked.

With a huff and a flurry, she jerked around and growled, "How do you think I did? What? Did you expect me to bomb? I'm a better writer than you are, Mom."

This was new. In the past, that same question would garner a lengthy explanation of how she aced the assignment and the clever manner in which she had done so. Not now. Discussing the changes in Chloe's behavior, Mark and I figured this might be a normal phase of adolescence since she was developing independence and taking on more responsibility. We had heard horror stories from friends with older children, chronicling painful stages of separation before leaving for college or career. I nudged back my worry by reflecting on those tales. But other concerns soon surfaced.

Chloe related details of arguments and disagreements with her friends and I often found it difficult to support, or even understand, her position. Her inability to get along with others spread beyond the walls of our home and negatively affected friendships. She displayed a sense of superiority, almost greatness that went beyond pride and into braggadocio. At times, her comments were embarrassing, judgmental, and even hateful.

One day she returned from school and smugly relayed the events of the day, "I let Kacie have it today. She struts around like she's better than everyone else, acting so righteous and judging the rest of us. At lunch, she was talking about Hannah behind her back, telling everybody she was giving guys blowjobs during vacation. So when I saw her in the hall between fifth and sixth hour, I yelled at her. I asked who she thought she was, talking about Hannah when she was having sex with Justin and screwed around with Daniel before him. I didn't know her sister was down the hall, but she heard everything. I hope she went home and told her mom. That'll teach her to talk crap."

Stunned by the unkind ruthlessness she had just recounted, I let out, "Chloe. You did this in front of other people? Why would you hurt Kacie like that? That's a terrible way to handle conflict with a friend."

"She deserved it. It was hilarious to see the look on her face. I hope her mom does find out."

Another incident with my mother further confirmed that something was terribly wrong with Chloe. My mom and Chloe had always had a close relationship, and when she visited, the two of them spent a lot of time together, chatting, sharing, and hanging out. One time Mom came to me, visibly concerned, when Chloe was not around.

"Do you know what Chloe said to me? I still can't believe it. She thinks the government should round up all the ugly people and all the stupid people and put them on their own island, so they don't pollute the gene pool. What's gotten into her? Where did she get such an idea? What makes her think it's okay to talk like that? I don't want to betray her confidence, but I think she needs a good talking to."

When I did talk to her, I got a half-hearted, "Oh, Mom, I was just messing around. Gram overreacted. But it's not a bad idea. It would accelerate natural selection." Chloe's callous lack of empathy stunned and disturbed me.

As her persona continued to change, it became rare for any activity involving Chloe to go smoothly, or as planned. The other kids expected her to create a scene or be demanding and difficult, and they no longer enjoyed her company. She was frequently late or unprepared, often changing her mind about participating at all. She still held her own at work, but slept through her alarm and arrived late a time or two. Conversations about the changes in her personality were impossible. She felt picked on and blamed. In all honesty, she was so demanding and hard to please, we probably did pick and blame. We felt relief when commitments kept her busy and away from home. When we were together, discord reigned. We enjoyed her company less and less.

I remember how difficult it was to get her senior pictures taken just weeks before school started. Already angry because I refused to buy new makeup for the session, she couldn't decide what to wear and wanted no assistance. We missed her appointment, but I called and the photographer was still willing to take her. Chloe was irritable and short-tempered as we got her un-ironed clothes together, and drove to the studio. Frazzled by the preceding fiasco, I had my fill when her angry attitude continued in the car. Halfway there, I pulled over.

"Chloe, I've had enough. You need to go to the photographer, but I don't have to be there and I will not allow you to treat me this way. I'm going home and you can go by yourself."

She burst into tears, shouting, "I can't believe you'd make me go by myself. This is a big day in my life and you act like it's a huge inconvenience. Most moms would be happy if their daughters wanted them to come, but not you. You just want me out of your way. You don't even care what's important to me."

Again, we had perceived the situation so differently. I figured she would be thrilled to get rid of me, but she panicked at the thought of being without me. Was it always this complicated for girls to separate from their mothers, and if so, how long would it last?

During the photo session, another interesting detail became apparent. Chloe had difficulty finding her smile. She could not come up with a natural smile. Now, this is common for three- to six-year-olds, but Chloe had never had difficulty performing for the camera. For most of her life, she would smile and strike a pose at the whirring sound of a warming flash feature. This was different. She seemed to have no control over her outward expression of emotion. My stomach churned as I watched, anxious. It took a long time for this experienced photographer to catch Chloe smiling naturally, and many of the proofs displayed surprising images. They reflected someone, but not our daughter.

Soon after that appointment, Chloe began dating a young man she had known for years. They worked together at the resort and spent a lot of time with each other outside of work hours. From the beginning it seemed an unsteady alliance, since this boy had a long-term girlfriend with whom he was still involved. Surprisingly, and against her usual value system, Chloe seemed not to care. She was smitten and enjoyed his company.

They had fun together and that was all that mattered. We talked about the obvious issues.

"Chloe, think about this. Taylor is still dating Angie. He obviously has feelings for her, and she'd be crushed if she knew you and Taylor were going out."

"I know Mom, but I really like him and we have fun together. Besides, I don't like Angie. I don't care if she gets hurt. She treats Taylor like crap most of the time."

"Well, if their relationship is falling apart give it the kind of respect you'd want if you were Angie. Wait until they break up before you go out with Taylor."

"I don't want to. I really like him."

"Why do you like him so much? What kind of character does he have if he's willing to deceive someone he says he loves? What does it say about your character if you're willing to be part of the deception?"

In some families, this conversation might seem invasive or unusual, but we had talked about values, morals, and ethics since the children were tiny. To Mark and I, personal integrity is a precious commodity. The very nature of this relationship was contrary to everything we had taught Chloe and assumed she valued. It became another strange piece in a rapidly emerging puzzle.

With great relief, we made it through the summer. In the fall of 1999, Chloe began her senior year taking five classes, editing the yearbook, and coaching Monica's soccer team. She still planned to work a few shifts a week to support an appreciation for shopping that went beyond the allowance we gave her. In fact, her spending surpassed her income too, as verified by a couple of bounced checks over the next few weeks. At times, she no longer saw the connection between wanting and earning, developing an egocentric sense of entitlement. She had a hard time keeping track of how much money she had and how much she spent. If she wanted something, it was worth the cost. This was a huge change from the budget-conscious teen that looked for bargains to stretch her clothing allowance.

Another big change was the void left in Chloe's social circle when many of her friends moved away to college. One of those friends was Taylor. She missed him terribly, and worried because he and Angie were attending the same university. Chloe became obsessed with Taylor and what he might be doing, wondering if he was coming to town for the weekend, or if he'd found a job near campus. She talked about him all the time and frequently called mutual friends to get the latest buzz. She felt profound loneliness. She missed the full and exciting summer routine and seemed bogged down by school and the demands of her busy schedule.

With fewer classes as a senior, Chloe did not start school until nearly nine o'clock each morning. The rest of us were up and running by six o'clock in the morning. Having grown accustomed to being alone in the house by about eight, I relished that quiet time, using it to write in my journal, read the paper, and organize my day before getting down to work. Now that quiet time was gone. During those morning hours, our home exploded into a battleground.

From her bed, Chloe shouted at Michael, "Turn your music down."

And at Monica, "Why can't you blow-dry your hair at night? I can't sleep."

She yelled at me if I used the blender or mixer while making breakfast, and screamed at all of us for opening and closing doors or talking to one another. Although she had never slept soundly, the problem had amplified in recent weeks. She awakened at the slightest noise. Tired, and furious at being aroused, she hurled insults and criticisms until Michael and Monica were out of the house. Shortly after they left, she would get up and get herself ready, with stereo and attitude blaring. I handled the situation poorly, engaging in head-to-head battle. Of course, I knew better. Creating a win/lose scenario is never a good idea for the mother of a teen. Palpable tension strained our relationship like never before.

Looking back at my journal, in mid-September 1999 I wrote: "I love her and I'm losing her and it makes me so sad. In sadness, I'm building walls and holding up hoops for her to jump through. I've become unlikable. She loves me but doesn't like me and sometimes the feeling is mutual. I exercise control and she wants that to stop. She says things and acts in ways she knows will hurt me. It's so unlike her. I admire and appreciate

her individuality, her spirit, and her potential, but I'm not
dealing well with any of them. She's changing radically and I
struggle to adapt to the changes."

A few days later, my journal verifies that Chloe was
beginning to fall into the abyss of depression: "Ahhggh. Last
night I sat with Chloe through a tearful, painful, talking-in-
circles discussion, trying to find the underlying cause of her
deep sadness. We grappled through layers of emotion to get to
the crux of the problem. It was so much work. She knows she
doesn't feel right, but can't put her feelings into words. She
wants me to help her, but I don't know how. I feel helpless and
frustrated, and at times angry at her inability to understand
herself, even though I know she would like nothing better than
to be more self-aware. Enlightenment seems inaccessible. As we
muddle   through,   we   learn   lessons   in   patience   and
communication, but what extreme effort. In the end she felt just
a little better and I was utterly drained."

As the weeks passed, my worry for Chloe grew. She no
longer awoke with the morning noise, but she did not awaken at
the sound of her alarm either. Many mornings, she was
physically unable to get out of bed. She sometimes slept through
entire days, only leaving her room to use the bathroom or get
something to eat. She would miss a few days of school, then
panic at the thought of falling behind, thus adding a thick layer
of anxiety to her depression. She eroded into a perpetually
shaking, tearful mass of emotion. I hardly recognized my oldest
child.

Then her depression exploded. It mushroomed. It devastated
her internal landscape and wrought havoc on every facet of her
life. She suffered. I tried to persuade her that this was not normal
and that she needed to go to the doctor. She saw it differently
and refused medical help. Her view: "This is me. You don't like
me. Why should I go to the doctor when the problem is that you
guys just don't like me?" This came from a child that we had
always adored. I was baffled.

In early October, I took Chloe to Dr. Sander, our family
doctor, for a follow-up visit to check her acne. While there, I told
Dr. Sander about Chloe's recent behavioral changes: the crying
jags, the anxiety, and sleep disturbances. Chloe was furious with

me for bringing it up. She glared, began to cry, and finally rebuked me in the controlled voice of someone who would like to shout but thinks better of it. She insisted it was none of my business and that I had no right to bring up her private affairs. I, too, cried, as I rationalized that my concerns for her well-being took precedence over my respect for her privacy. No matter what I said, Chloe had a response and grew more adamant in her disapproval. Throughout this heated exchange, Dr. Sander listened and observed. Then she stood up and shared her opinions.

"Chloe, it's clear that you're dealing with some pretty serious depression. I know you don't like the idea that something might be wrong with you, but this is not your normal behavior. I understand that you're angry with your mom for telling me, but she's worried, and rightfully so. I'm writing you a prescription for Prozac, and giving you the names of counselors I refer my patients to. I never put teenagers on anti-depressants without counseling, too."

Dr. Sander speculated that Chloe would require six to twelve months of medication along with regular counseling sessions to help her identify triggers and develop behavioral changes. "I see this more often than you'd believe, especially in high-achieving students. You'll feel a lot better in a few weeks."

When we left Dr. Sander's office Chloe was still furious, but I felt as if we were on the right track. I filled her prescription, made an appointment with a counselor, and looked through some pamphlets about depression and its treatment.

After reading the information the doctor provided, I wondered if I, too, might need an anti-depressant. I realized then that I thought depression was something we overcame through strength of character and willpower. I feared that I had tainted my daughter, allowing her to develop unhealthy perceptions of herself. Through example, I had sent the erroneous message that mental health was an individual responsibility, and that a person's inability to "get a grip" was a personal failure. Here I took my first step on the erroneous path of martyrdom, assuming that Chloe's well-being was my responsibility.

Seeing depression in my daughter rather than in the mirror softened my heart. I grew less critical. After reading several books on the topic, I realized that I had had chronic depression since early childhood and recognized the strategies and coping mechanisms I employed over the years in order to "be okay." I began to understand depression's biological roots, and consider treatment options. I shared my newfound knowledge and attitudes with Mark, and we hoped that Chloe would soon feel better.

4

October 1999

"... then black despair
The shadow of a starless night, was thrown
Over the world in which I move alone..."
  —Percy Bysshe Shelley

Our hopes for a quick and easy cure vanished. After five weeks on medication, Chloe's depression deepened. She no longer had an interest in attending school or going to work and was not fulfilling her yearbook obligations or going to soccer practices. She rarely got out of her pajamas or showered. As her mental state deteriorated, I tried to cheer her up, tried to convince her that it was not that bad. However, my inner alarms blared.

One afternoon, following another missed day of school, Chloe said, "Mom, what if something worse is happening to me? What if I have what Grandma had?" This was the first time any of us drew a parallel between Chloe's situation and her grandmother's rarely discussed mental illness. Out of ignorance or fear, I pooh-poohed the idea, telling her she would feel better soon. Then I made one of the biggest mistakes of my life.

"We can fix this, Chloe. It just takes time," I told her. "It's not as if you hear voices or see things that aren't real, like Grandma did. It's not that bad. Don't worry."

To this day, those are the words I would most like to take back, the comments I most deeply regret.

A few nights later, feeling both depressed and anxious, Chloe went into the kitchen for a glass of lemonade. Struggling with constantly shaking hands, she dropped the glass and jumped, landing on a glass shard. She began to cry, and melted to the floor, one of her toes nearly severed. We tightly wrapped the foot and Mark helped her to the car while I got my things together for a trip to the emergency room. Mark stayed with Michael and Monica, and Chloe and I went to the hospital. She sobbed during the entire ride.

Once at the emergency room, I put Chloe in a wheelchair, registered her, and then parked my car. She was still crying when I returned, but said her foot didn't hurt. As we waited in a treatment room for a doctor to stitch her up, the crying finally stopped. A short time later, her demeanor frightened me. Her affect went flat. Her eyes went blank, her face lax, and she would not speak. A chill of fear sliced through my core. I recognized this state. I had seen Mark's mom, Elizabeth, languish in and out of it for years.

As a nurse scrubbed the wounded foot and gave Chloe a tetanus shot and the doctor stitched her up, she did not react. She seemed oblivious to discomfort despite what was going on. I was shocked, because Chloe has a low tolerance for pain and no problem letting you know when something hurt. While we were in that emergency room, I thought about her general health and knew the Prozac was not working. Chloe was worse. Terror blazed a trail through me. We went back to the doctor the next day.

This time Dr. Sander asked more questions about family history, trying to get a better handle on how to treat Chloe's depression. She asked about members of our extended family whose depression improved with treatment, and I told her my mom took Zoloft with good results. With a link of success established, the doctor wrote a Zoloft prescription for Chloe and, as I finally confided my own history of depression to her, she wrote another one for me. I could no longer keep myself together and help my daughter, too.

Blessedly, the Zoloft did the trick for me. Within two or three weeks, I felt the cloud of depression lift and was amazed by the relative ease of each day. I no longer had to work hard to maintain my mood. It surprised me, really, and I began to understand that this was how most people lived and felt. I joked with Mark about how easy he had it. It was not "normal" to struggle for contentedness the way I always had, and now I felt liberated. From my earliest memories, a sense of well-being required my focused effort. Suddenly now, that internal exertion was no longer necessary. Taking an anti-depressant for the rest of my life was a small price to pay to enjoy this previously elusive sense of balance. I was elated.

One journal entry reads: "I notice a clearness of thought and peace of mind that I have never before experienced. Is it possible that, with medication, I can feel this sense of well-being all the time? Depression has robbed me of so much joy, contributed such anxiety to my life. I had no idea."

Despite the challenges with Chloe's health, I felt so good. My life's new potential excited me. Now I understood the havoc a chemical imbalance in the brain can create in a person's body, a person's life. Unfortunately, Chloe did not respond similarly. She now slept with Mark and me, or on the floor next to my side of the bed. She awakened in a panic several times a night, settling down only after I held her hands and rubbed her head and shoulders to soothe her back to sleep. During the day, she laid in bed or near me, unable to do the simplest tasks. She did not go to school and no longer kept up in her classes.

Listless but still eating regularly, Chloe gained weight, adding to her despair. She panicked if I was not in sight or earshot. However, most concerning, she constantly battled suicidal thoughts, or ideations, despite taking the medication and seeing her therapist, Maria, once a week. Fortunately, she talked about the thoughts swirling in her mind but did not act on them. I took her back to Dr. Sander, who admitted that Chloe's depression was out of her league. She recommended we find a psychiatrist.

I spent hours on the phone to find a psychiatrist who would take a seventeen-year-old. Her age was problematic. Adult psychiatrists would not see her, and child psychiatrists either did not want to take a patient so close to age eighteen, or were not taking new patients. I finally got an appointment, but it was weeks away.

5

November 1999

"The diseases of the mind are more and more destructive than those of the body."
— Marcus Tullius Cicero

My regular routine turned inside out. After years of volunteering at the local Cooperative Extension Office, I gave up my position to be at home with Chloe. My shifts were interrupted by her distressed phone calls or cut short when I left to make sure she was safe. Because I was no longer reliable, it was time to call it quits.

At home, I worked on the book I was writing while Chloe rested on a nearby sofa. On bad days, she lay on the floor next to my chair where we could maintain physical contact. She was missing so much and I constantly worried about how to get her back on track as quickly as possible. As much as I wanted her life back to normal, I yearned for my own freedom and independence, too. I resented the loss, and then felt ashamed for feeling resentful. I reminded myself that Chloe did not ask for this to happen, it was not her choice or her fault. I struggled with my own storm of emotions.

Feeling trapped and frustrated one morning, I tried to get away for a cup of coffee with my good friend, Tina. I told Chloe where I was going and when I would be back. The coffee shop was only five minutes from the house and I had my cell phone in case panic threatened to overwhelm her. Just hearing my voice often calmed her down and kept the anxiety from growing unbearable. I thought she could manage for a short time without me, but after only ten minutes, she phoned.

"Mom," she croaked through sobs and heaving breaths, "I want you to come home. I'm afraid. I don't feel right. I don't know what's wrong. Please come home. I don't want to be by myself."

Irritated that I could not be away, even briefly, I snapped. "Chloe, I'm five minutes away. You know where I am and you will be fine. I'm going to sit here and drink my coffee and then I'll be home. I think you can handle being alone for that short time."

I felt manipulated and questioned, as I often had these past few weeks, whether I was overindulging her or she was this ill. She cried and begged some more, but I stood my ground and told her I'd be home soon before saying goodbye and getting off the phone. Ten minutes later, my phone rang again.

"Kate, this is Maria. I just got off the phone with Chloe and she is upset. You need to go home immediately. I don't think you understand how fragile she is. She's in real danger of hurting herself and absolutely cannot be left alone."

I told Tina I had to leave and ran out of the coffee shop. I don't know what was more sobering: the anger at losing control of my own life, the shame I felt for putting my daughter's life at risk, or the fact that I'd been called on it. Regardless, that moment spawned great change.

When I got home, I found Chloe sitting on the edge of her bed, the phone at her ear with Maria on the other end. I took the phone, assured Maria that I would remain with Chloe, and then hung up. Chloe rocked back and forth, wracked by breathtaking sobs, for several hours until her body gave up and she fell asleep. After that, we began to live our lives around Chloe's illness, even canceling plans to go to a family wedding in favor of keeping things calm and remaining close to her therapist. Those changes turned out to be wise.

Late one evening I awoke to light beneath my bedroom door and unusual noises emanating from the family room. I got up to investigate and encountered Chloe in the clutches of what I later learned was a severe manic episode. She leaned against the back of the sofa in what looked like a standing fetal position. Her toes curled under and her feet turned in at the ankles, reminding me of Chinese women after years of torturous foot binding.

Her knees, shoulders, and elbows bent slightly, creating the profile of someone very old. Both hands pulled into her chest, claw like, and so tightly twisted that her fingernails cut into the skin on the palms of her hands. Her head tilted forward, hair covering her face. Her entire body was rigid and trembling at the same time, and she not only sobbed, but also made a hissing sound. The most alarming element was her facial expression, so contorted that it frightened me. I began to cry, too.

I lifted Chloe's head to look into her face, and her eyes rolled back. Her head shook so vigorously, spittle flew off her chin and splattered on my forearms. She continued to hiss through tightly clenched teeth. I remember thinking this was like a scene from a film. Surreal now had meaning for me. Ridiculously, I tried to get her to talk, peppering her with questions, petting her head, and eroding into my own state of panic.

We made such a racket that Mark and Michael woke up and came into the family room. "Mark, I don't know what's going on," I sobbed. "I don't know what to do. I'm not sure she can hear me. It's like she's not in there."

When, after several minutes, we failed to get a coherent response from Chloe, we knew we had to get her to the hospital. The three of us maneuvered her into the garage and then the backseat of the car, but not before a true miracle occurred. As we prepared to move her, Chloe seemed herself for mere seconds — just long enough to raise her head, look into my eyes, and whisper through clenched teeth, "Mommy, I'm still in here."

That was the first of many incidents that kept my fear from overwhelming me, and allowed me to maintain hope. Throughout our ordeal, similar experiences have intensified my faith, magnified my love for Chloe, and verified that we would learn life-altering, soul-changing lessons as we figured this out together. Without that moment, feelings of fear and helplessness might have overcome my love and determination to fight for my child. However, that miraculous occurrence galvanized my faith and encouraged me.

Mark drove while I sat in back with Chloe. Michael stayed home with Monica. We arrived at the hospital near midnight. Mark and I lifted Chloe into a wheelchair, since by this time she had no motor control. We discovered that a person who looks out of her mind garners a lot of attention, and we received immediate help. I told the admitting nurse that Chloe was taking Zoloft for depression, and they contacted the on-call psychiatrist who was already in the building. The doctor quickly injected Chloe with Ativan for what he told us was an acute anxiety-laden reaction to the Zoloft. He cautioned us not to let her take any more Zoloft and to get her into a psychiatrist as soon as possible. We waited several hours as the medication took effect and her body and mind returned to a near normal, although exhausted, state.

Mark and I were exhausted, too, and the ramifications of what we had experienced tumbled around in our minds. We were frightened, dumbfounded, and emotionally off-balance. For the first time we both considered that our child might be afflicted with a serious mental illness. Could Chloe and his mom have the same diagnosis? We'd never discussed the topic. It was taboo. Surprisingly, we did not talk much about it then. It was too sad a possibility. We just wanted to get Chloe home, and when we did, she slept and slept.

She slept, that is, until nausea woke her up. Then she vomited, trembled, ached, and hardly slept for three full days. I phoned the hospital and they put me in touch with the staff psychiatrist in the children's ward of the affiliated psychiatric hospital. He told me that Chloe's reaction was the predictable result of suddenly stopping the Zoloft, which is a selective serotonin reuptake inhibitor. Her brain now had a precariously low level of accessible serotonin, a chemical vital to mood and well-being. Oddly, this deficiency produced flu-like symptoms, including nausea, muscle aches, and extreme fatigue. In addition, her system was dealing with an excessive amount of Ativan, which contributed to headache, dizziness, and poor equilibrium. She was experiencing physical sensations similar to those that an alcoholic suffers when he stops drinking, cold turkey.

I was furious that nobody told us this could happen, and felt helpless because there was nothing we could do to help her through it. I began to develop an intimate familiarity with the lack of control that accompanies caring for a loved one with a chronic illness.

Several days later when the dizziness and nausea abated, and she was strong enough to endure a car ride, I took Chloe to see Maria. Ordinarily, I accompanied her to Maria's office and read a book in the waiting room, joining them for the last few minutes. Sometimes, if I had obligations with Michael or Monica, I'd drop Chloe off and pick her up later, and then Maria would call and fill me in. Of course, Chloe always knew what we talked about, and from the very beginning no conversation or decision-making took place without her complete involvement or consent.

This time the routine was different. Only a few minutes into their session, Maria wanted to talk to me. She didn't think Chloe had a simple case of depression. Based on previous sessions with Chloe, and after hearing about our most recent hospital ordeal, Maria wondered if Chloe might suffer from hypomania (which, I later learned, was a sub-type of Bipolar Disorder). I had never heard of it. She gave us some basic information regarding the illness and explained why she thought it was likely. Then she did a wonderful thing. She called the psychiatric hospital and asked, as a colleague, to speak to the doctor on staff. Within minutes, Chloe had an appointment to see him at the hospital the next morning. We were getting somewhere.

Before we left her office, Maria also told me, step by step, how to admit Chloe to the hospital if that was necessary to keep her from hurting herself before we saw the doctor in the morning. Again, I was shocked and ashamed by my inability fully to recognize the gravity of my child's condition. Even after everything that had happened I did not know that she was in imminent peril.

This "not knowing" was particularly difficult for me to reconcile with my perceptions of myself as a mother and a compassionate person. I'd committed myself to full-time parenting. I was "doing it right." I prided myself on being tuned in to my children's needs. This disconnect from the reality of my child's situation challenged my elemental sense of self. I thought, "By allowing Chloe to get this sick without realizing the seriousness, I've proven that I'm not the person I thought I was." Then my esteem dropped lower ... "I am not a good mother," ... and to the very lowest, "I am not good."

I went to bed but did not sleep. Thoughts of inadequacy and then rationalization swam through my mind. I mentally dissected the events leading up to Maria's earlier comments, starting as far back as Chloe's early childhood. I wondered about her fussy infancy and disinterest in playing with other children when she was a child. I particularly focused on a conversation we had when she was about ten. After finishing homework, Michael went out to rollerblade with the neighborhood kids and Monica was busy creating an elaborate Barbie town. Chloe tailed me as I finished my housekeeping and prepared dinner.

"Chloe, why don't you want to rollerblade with the other kids?" I asked, wondering why following me around the house was more fun than playing outdoors.

"No. I don't want to. I'd rather stay inside."

"Would you like to invite Brianne over? She has called almost every day to see if you want to play. Doesn't that sound like fun?"

"No. I see her at school all the time. I don't want to see her at home, too."

"Okay then. How about Kathy? You always have fun with her, and she's right across the street. Go see if she wants to ride bikes or jump on the trampoline."

"Mom, I don't want to be around other kids. I don't really like it."

"What do you mean, you 'don't really like it'?"

"It's hard. It's too much work to be with other people. It's not worth it. I have to do that all day at school and I don't want to do it when I get home. I'd rather be with you or by myself."

Baffled by that response, I didn't know how to react.

I remember being concerned about Chloe's social skills at that time. Both her second- and third-grade teachers wanted to skip a grade and I refused. I feared she'd have trouble socializing in a classroom of older children. I already worried about that facet of her life. Memories flooded back and I wondered why I had not sought professional help then. However, I reminded myself, she got good grades, was well mannered, and seemed happy. Even though she did not want to play with other children, she had friends and never had conflicts. While of concern, her comments that day seemed more idiosyncratic that pathogenic.

I spent the rest of the night similarly analyzing her childhood, searching for clues that I felt I should have noticed, precursors to recent events. I beat myself up for what I never knew.

6
Mid-November 1999

"Which of the mes is me?
The wild, impulsive, chaotic, energetic, and crazy one?
Or the shy, withdrawn, desperate, suicidal, doomed and tired one?"
  — Kay Redfield Jamison

We saw Dr. Kahil the next morning. He had already conferenced with Maria and proceeded to ask Chloe and me about the past few months. Then he probed further, asking about her birth, early childhood experiences and illnesses, high school years, and recent events. Some of the topics surprised me because they pinpointed behaviors and situations that had concerned me over the years, including many of the scenarios I had walked through during my sleepless night. However, I had to admit, I had never linked those incidents to mental illness … until then.

After taking the medical history of pregnancy and delivery, Dr. Kahil wanted to know more about Chloe.

"What kind of baby was she? Was she fussy, or generally content?"

I honestly told him how difficult she had been as an infant. "She cried a lot, but I could settle her down. And then something else would make her cry. That lasted until she was about six months old and began to crawl. But," I added, "she was really bright. She reached developmental milestones much earlier than normal."

"How did she respond to changes in her environment when she was very young?"

"Oh my gosh. That was the problem. Every little change was more than she could tolerate. If it got cold, she cried. If it got hot, she cried. If the lighting changed, she cried."

At this point in the conversation Chloe chimed in with, "Wow, things haven't changed much have they, Mom? I still can't stand it if I get too hot or too cold, and I'm always too hot or too cold."

This was true. We often joked that Chloe had a comfort zone that spanned all of four degrees.

Dr. Kahil asked me to continue.

"She got hysterical in stores with lots of fluorescent lighting and could hardly tolerate crowded rooms or a lot of noise." Then I smiled and told him about the conversation I had had with her sweet pediatrician seventeen years earlier.

He smiled back. "Sounds like you had a good pediatrician." He peppered me with more questions. "Did she eat often?"

"Every three hours until she was six months old, and then it began to normalize."

"Did she sleep well? Awaken frequently? Suffer from sleep disturbances?"

Again, I was flabbergasted at how his questions seemed to hone in on Chloe's habits. "She didn't sleep through the night until she was three years old, and still had night terrors several times a week until she was five or six. Even now, she sleeps poorly. If I think about it, I guess she never developed good, solid sleep patterns."

Then I recalled and shared a particular conversation I had had with my sister-in-law, an educator with a Master's degree in early childhood development, and the mother of three children herself. She'd said, "You know, Kate, if Chloe had been my first child, I would never have had another. She was one of the most difficult babies I'd ever encountered. It was so hard to keep her happy, and she never slept. I don't know how you did it."

"But," I told the doctor, "the other side of the coin was equally dramatic. As much as she cried, Chloe smiled more than any baby I had ever been around, and she was determined to talk, to use language to make her wants known. Sights and sounds fascinated her, and she mimicked them when she was tiny. She loved it when we held her and read to her, sang to her and talked to her, played with her and took her for walks. When she wasn't fussy, she was exceptionally happy."

"Did she develop language early?"

"Oh yeah. She really did communicate in complete sentences well before she was two. She's always been unusually articulate. In grade school, her language skills were precocious. When people first met her they often commented that she sounded like an adult. One of her babysitters," I continued, "told me she had the soul of a very old woman."

He smiled again, and so did Chloe.

"Did she show signs of separation anxiety, or get really upset if you left?"

"She had difficulty with that for years."

"What do you mean 'had'?" Chloe asked. "I still feel really anxious when I know you're not going to be around."

Then we told him about my recent trip to the coffee shop and the subsequent phone calls from Chloe and Maria, and Chloe tried to explain the physical sensations she experienced when she felt that kind of anxiety.

"I feel like I'm coming out of my skin, like my body can't contain my insides. My heart pounds and I shake all over. It's hard to catch my breath. Thoughts start going through my mind so quickly, I can hardly recognize them, and then they fly through again, round and round. Scary thoughts. Bad thoughts. Or maybe they're feelings not thoughts, I don't know. I feel like I'm not safe, like I'm in danger. Like an animal when it knows a predator is near."

I had not heard this before and felt terrible about my lack of understanding. I had misunderstood, underestimated, the degree of discomfort and fear she experienced.

Dr. Kahil nodded his head, seeming to recognize the sensations Chloe described. He moved on, asking about her relationships with peers and schoolmates, which, as I had reminded myself the night before, had always been less intense, less significant, than I had observed in students during my years as an elementary school teacher.

"What about academics?"

"She's brilliant," I told him. "When she was in fourth grade her teacher told me that Chloe was smarter than he was. Two other teachers wanted to skip a grade, but I refused because I didn't want her to struggle socially. She didn't interact with other children the way I thought she should. She often isolated herself, declined invitations to parties and other fun activities. She frequently told me that it was 'too hard' to play with other kids, too much work."

As I spoke the words aloud, I realized that Chloe had constructed her own, quiet routine even in early childhood.

He asked about Chloe's sexual activity, and drug and alcohol use. He wanted to know if she'd ever been violent or hurt anyone. Her answers affirmed that she was a good kid. She tried hard to please us, had a strong sense of right and wrong, and wanted to live up to that. I found out later that we were very lucky in this arena. Most teenagers diagnosed with her illness experiment with drugs and alcohol in an effort to assuage the discomfort they feel. Many of them become addicted, promiscuous, or violent.

Then Dr. Kahil delved into our family medical histories. Going back several generations, my family tree was laden with alcoholism, drug abuse, depression, and suicide. Mark's family was much more private about health and other personal issues, but we knew his mom suffered from a serious mental illness. For years she had taken numerous prescriptions, including antidepressants, anti-psychotics, and anti-anxiety medications.

Several times in the last decade of her life, she had spent weeks at a time in the psychiatric ward at a local hospital. She sometimes suffered from delusions and paranoia, thinking people around her had committed crimes, and even refused to eat for lengthy periods because she thought someone was trying to poison her. For years she was so heavily medicated she barely functioned at all, sleeping most of the time, and rarely conversing when she was awake. I thought she was probably schizophrenic, but no one talked about it. No one questioned it. No one shared information.

Then Dr. Kahil directed his attention to Chloe and she answered him honestly and frankly. "Describe the sensations you feel when you're depressed."

"My body feels too heavy to move. I just want to sleep, or at least lie down all the time. My brain doesn't work right either. It's like I'm thinking through thick fog. Everything is slow and heavy. The worst part is I just don't want to do anything. I have no motivation."

"Tell me about your current sleep habits."

"I sleep all the time during the day because I don't sleep at night. I don't like to sleep at night. I can only sleep if I know my mom is right there. I get scared."

"Do you have vivid, violent, or gory nightmares?"

She began to cry.

"Yes. I see things in my mind that are really bad, violent, scary. Someone is always getting hurt, or just about to get hurt when I wake up. Sometimes I see the scary stuff when I'm dreaming, but sometimes it seems like I see them when I'm not asleep. I can't always remember the difference between things I dream, or see on television, or things I think about, and things I really did. Sometimes I'm not sure if things really happened or not."

"Do you hear voices or see things that aren't really there?"

Chloe looked down at her feet, then back up at my face, tears streaming down her splotchy, red cheeks.

Dr. Kahil pressed. "That question made you uncomfortable. Do you hear voices or see thing that aren't really there?" he asked again.

"No. I'm not crazy."

"I don't think you're crazy, Chloe. I think you have an illness and I'm trying to figure out what it is. The more you tell me, and honestly, the better chance I have of figuring this out. So, do you ever have voices in your head, or get ideas that make you want to do something you know you shouldn't do?"

"Sometimes."

"Tell me about that."

"I don't want to. I don't want my mom to know how bad I am."

I forced back my tears. "Chloe, I don't think you're bad. You've always been a good girl. This isn't your fault. You've done nothing wrong. Tell us everything that's happening so the doctor and Maria and Daddy and I can help you get better."

"But what if I don't get better? I don't want to be like that. I'd rather die."

"Do you think about killing yourself?" Dr. Kahil asked. "Have you thought about how you'd do that?"

"I think about it a lot, but I don't know how I'd do it. I don't want my mom or my brother and sister to find me. I thought about crashing my truck, but I don't want to ruin it. Mostly, I just see myself gone, dead, and wish that were how it was. I'd like to go to sleep and not wake up. I just want to be done."

"Well," said Dr. Kahil, "I want you to promise right now that you won't do anything to hurt yourself, or do anything that might make you die. I can help you get better, but I can't do that if you hurt yourself. Do you understand me?"

"Yes."

"Do you promise that you won't try to take your own life and that if the temptation becomes overwhelming, you'll tell your mom?"

"I won't do anything. I'll tell my mom."

"Good, Chloe. Now Mrs. McLaughlin, do you know how to check Chloe into the hospital if she's a danger to herself or others?"

"Maria explained the process to me yesterday in case Chloe got worse before we had our appointment with you."

"Okay. If you have to admit her to the hospital, I want you to let them know that I'm her psychiatrist. I'm the chief on the pediatric ward and they contact me immediately when one of my patients comes in. Chloe, do you ever hurt yourself, but not really badly, and without intending to kill yourself?"

"No. Not really."

"Okay then. Do you think it's possible that something might not be working right in your brain?"

"Oh, I know it."

After about an hour of these candid questions and answers, Dr. Kahil told us that he was certain that Chloe had Bipolar Disorder.

(For information on juvenile onset bipolar disorder, visit the Juvenile Bipolar Research Foundation website at www.jbrf.org)

7

Late November 1999

"By our own spirits are we deified;
We Poets in our youth begin in gladness;
But thereof comes in the end despondency and madness."
   —William Wordsworth

After dropping that Bipolar bomb on us, Dr. Kahil spent a fair amount of time on the topic of managing the illness with medication, therapy, and lifestyle changes. He gave us pamphlets about serious mental illness in general, and Bipolar Disorder in particular. He wrote a prescription for Depakote, explained the initial effects and side effects it might have on Chloe, and asked if we had any questions. Reeling from shock, I could think of nothing to ask. With that, Dr. Kahil asked to see Chloe in a week, and told us to call if we needed anything in the meantime.

I felt like we were communicating in a foreign language. I did not understand much of what he said, and did not want to hear the rest. My mind struggled to grasp the seriousness of the situation and my heart yearned to protect my child from the inevitable. My stomach churned. My heart pounded. I broke out in a sweat and felt chilled at the same time. I fought to catch my breath, sighing deeply several times before I breathed normally again. I was not sure if I was happy to have a diagnosis and a treatment plan, or if I wanted to pretend none of this was happening. I now understood why Mark's family did their best to ignore the reality of his mother's illness. It's just so big.

I barely absorbed the details of that meeting. For a few days, I felt like I had stopped dead in my tracks. I slept little, cried often, and prayed a lot. Fear gripped me as I imagined the horrible possibilities that could face Chloe, could face us. Now that we knew we were dealing with a chronic and often devastating mental illness, the grieving began. I felt like I had lost a child, even though Chloe was alive, if not well. I had many expectations for her, expectations for her future, her life, and our life. I lamented that those expectations would remain unfulfilled.

Chloe, Mark, and I mourned the loss of normalcy, the loss of health. All five of us felt the emotional burden and disappointment that every patient with a chronic illness feels, that every family member of a sick child or sibling endures. I doubted myself, wondering what I had done wrong, either physically or emotionally, to make this happen. I beat myself up and then I turned on God, wondering what in heaven's name He thought He was doing. I cried myself to sleep and Chloe did, too. Mark did his best to comfort and encourage us. Michael and Monica did their best to lay low, and Chloe and I sunk a little lower for a while, thinking about the changes this could bring.

Then we moved on to the next stage of grief. I got into "fix-it" mode and Chloe became more determined. She got back to studies and I hit the Internet, ordering every book available on the subject. I browsed every Website dedicated to Bipolar Disorder or mental illness. It was as if I was back in graduate school, working on a thesis. I would not battle this dangerous foe unarmed. Knowledge and information became my weapons of choice. I mustered my faith and my confidence and decided that we could handle this.

I figured I had two paths to follow. I could disengage and leave Chloe's illness and healthcare to her, or I could become proactive, leading the march toward creating a better life for her, for us. Thus began my quest to read and understand everything I could get my hands on regarding Bipolar Disorder, its history, current treatments, and my daughter's potential for a happy, productive future.

By this time, we'd reached the last few weeks of the semester. Chloe had already dropped her Pre-Calculus/ Trigonometry class because the Depakote rendered her unable to do the math problems that she had previously managed with ease. We learned that drugs used to treat mental illness, like medications for many chronic ailments, change not only the chemical and electrical impulses that lead to illness, but other parts of the brain as well, sometimes inexplicably.

Chloe was enrolled in four classes. She no longer worked or coached soccer. She desperately wanted to finish the semester without incompletes, so I made it my goal to get her to and from school every day and get her assignments turned in. We explained the situation to her teachers and they agreed not to lower her marks due to absences. Each of them was willing to base her semester grade solely on the work that was required and turned in.

Her amazing intellect and determined spirit shined brightly during this time as she completed the work she'd missed, took final exams, and ended up with two A's and two B's. As thrilled as I was with this achievement, Chloe was devastated. She had been an all-A student, and was angry that this illness had pounced, trying to devour what she prized the most—her mind.

Though she performed beautifully at school, Chloe's health grew worse instead of better. The Depakote caused weight gain and made her skin break out worse than ever. These two issues, combined with anxiety and depression, created a miserable creature. She cried unprovoked, then cried because she did not know why she was crying. She couldn't focus or remember, and was plagued by fear and paranoia, especially at night. Her nightmares increased in frequency and gore, so she didn't want to sleep. She grew so dependant on me, I even left the bathroom door open when I went in. This dependence took its toll.

I rarely saw anyone other than family and healthcare providers. On those infrequent occasions when I got together with my friend, Tina, she usually commented on how bad my eyes looked. "Your eyes tell everything I need to know, Kate. I can see into your soul. I'm as worried about you as you are about Chloe. Is it not getting better?"

"It'll get better soon. It has to."

Dr. Kahil assured us it would take a few weeks for the medication to reach optimal levels in Chloe's system.

"I know it's hard, but you have to be patient. She will get better, but it takes time. This illness traumatizes the brain. You can liken it to a physical injury. It takes a while for medications to put an end to that ongoing trauma, and even longer for the brain to heal."

I called my family and canceled Christmas plans. Mark took time off and we spent two weeks at home together. We were exhausted. We were not up to dealing with anybody else, were not ready to reveal what was going on. We were content to recuperate from the trauma of the past few weeks.

8
December 1999

"The loving personality seeks not to control, but to nurture, not to dominate, but to empower. Love is the richness and fullness of your soul flowing through you."
—Gary Zukav

Looking back at my journal and photographs from that holiday season, our exhaustion, fear, determination, and hope shine through. Although we had enjoyed years of wonderful holiday seasons filled with fond memories, this particular year, despite the challenges, we internalized the true meaning of Christmas and developed a deeper, more realistic appreciation of one another and the blessings we shared. A jumble of emotions that often seemed incongruent replaced our usual holiday fervor. We knew that being alive and together were precious gifts, but we were distraught because of the realities that made this clear. Coming to terms with Chloe's diagnosis sapped Mark's and my energy. At night, we would lie in bed and talk about what it meant.

"I can hardly think of anything else," I told him repeatedly, as we huddled together beneath the covers. "My mind is focused on learning everything I can about Bipolar Disorder, figuring out the best treatments, and adjusting our life to suit her needs. And then I feel guilty because I don't know how to balance it all and give Monica and Michael everything they need, too."

Mark proved, time after time, to be the calming voice of reason.

"We'll figure it out. There isn't a kid in the world whose every need is met all the time. We'll take care of them as we always have. They'll be okay."

I hoped he was right.

We reduced our normally hectic holiday schedule, avoiding parties and trips to the mall. We shared good meals made up of favorite dishes, watched movies, built jigsaw puzzles, competed in card games, and tried to understand and support one another. Monica and Michael asked few questions about Chloe's health, but when they did, Mark and I answered truthfully without too much detail. We didn't want to scare them, but didn't want to hide anything either.

Chloe did not interact with us as she normally would. She spent more time in her room and talked very little. If I sat on the sofa to watch a movie, she would lie down with her head in my lap and watch, too. She went to bed in her room most nights, but usually ended up in ours. A few times, she even crawled into bed with one of the other children. She saw no friends, talked to no one on the phone, and made no effort to leave the house, much less get out of her pajamas.

My journal for 30 December 1999 reads: "Chloe has not gotten better. In fact, her illness is much more severe than any of us realized. Ironically, she's doing so well, considering the obstacles. Unbeknownst to all of us, she's managed to overcome a severe mental illness for quite some time and has continued to perform exceptionally well at school and at home. I couldn't be more proud of her. I couldn't be more impressed with her determination to achieve and succeed, to overcome."

Chloe's depression deepened, and in some ways, with good reason. The medication she took had a long list of worrisome side effects, some potentially life threatening, requiring her to submit to blood work every couple of weeks. Nevertheless, the two less-medically challenging side effects — weight gain and worsening acne — were unbearable for her. After five years under a doctor's care to keep acne under control, the current Depakote-driven outbreak shattered her self-esteem. Most of her clothes were now too small, and she despaired when the new things we picked up were two sizes larger than she had ever worn. Even if the medication was working on the chemical causes of her illness, the physical effects seemed counter-productive, leaving her in worse shape than before. She avoided all of the activities her friends planned. Since she always declined invitations, they called less often.

Around that time, none of us followed normal routines or saw close friends. When Mark had the chance to go to his once-quarterly poker game, I practically pushed him out the door. He had enjoyed very little entertainment or relaxation in the past few months. He put in long hours and shouldered a great many responsibilities at work. He was an exceptional provider, and a wonderful husband and father. As Chloe's illness worsened, Mark assumed more household responsibilities and was as exhausted as I was by the challenges.

On that particular night, things were calm at home and the children and I were tired, planning an early bedtime. Around ten o'clock I checked on them. They were all asleep. I unplugged the Christmas lights, put our new puppy in his cubby, and got ready for bed. I was reading before turning out the light when Chloe's friend, Jade, telephoned. The unusually late call surprised and delighted me. The girls had not gotten together recently and I hoped Chloe was awake and would take the call. I asked Jade to hold on and carried the phone across the house to Chloe's room. No light was visible under her door, so I gently knocked to see if she would respond. Hearing a slight rustle, I opened the door. Opening that door was like opening Pandora's Box, and I was unprepared for what emerged.

Tightly rolled towels lay snugly against the bottom of the bedroom's double doors, preventing light from shining out. Contrary to its earlier—and of late, normal—condition, the bedroom was spotless. Everything was in its rightful place. Drawers were shut, the closet closed, and for the first time in weeks, the bed was made. Adding welcome yet incongruent warmth, a candle glowed softly atop a corner shelf. In the center of this right and tidy room, Chloe sat on a towel, spread on the floor to keep her blood from ruining the carpet, slowly and methodically cutting her wrist with a razor.

"What the hell are you doing?"

Within seconds I hung up on Jade, ran to Chloe, who was still cutting, and took the razor from her hand. Blood covered her forearm and thigh. Small pieces of precious white flesh clung to the razor's edge. She was giving up. I was frightened and angry. I raised the bleeding wrist above her head, tightly wrapping it with one of the towels near the door, and began to cry. I looked squarely into her face. She stared back through glassy, unfocused eyes set in profound and utter sadness. I saw her soul laid bare, caught a glimpse of her deep pain and disillusionment. I will be forever grateful that Jade called. I am convinced that call saved Chloe's life.

Keeping Chloe's arm above her head, I removed the towel to assess the severity of the injury. I must have interrupted her shortly after she'd begun to cut, because the wound was somewhat superficial. Still holding her arm above her head, I led Chloe into the bathroom and sat her on the floor. Then I washed her wrist, butterflied the gaping flesh, and wrapped it in a gauze bandage. The wrist probably needed stitches, but I was afraid of a mandatory stay in the Psych Ward after a suicide attempt, so didn't even consider taking her to the hospital. Of course, if her wounds were truly life threatening, I would have taken her in a heartbeat, but I figured I could patch her up and take care of her at home. Irrationally, I did not want a psychiatric hospitalization in her medical records. Functioning from a position of stigma and shame that is still all too common, I wanted to keep our ordeal as private as possible.

Through it all, Chloe did not fight me, did not talk, and did not respond. When we were finished, she raised her face to mine and stated matter-of-factly, "Next time I'll cut the other way, straight down the vein. It'll be faster and you won't be able to fix it."

We had taken another turn on this rapid, downward spiral of insanity.

After I finished bandaging her arm, I searched Chloe's bedroom and the bathrooms, removing everything I thought she could use to hurt herself. As I went through drawers and boxes, her affect remained flat, emotionless. While I was in her closet, she began to giggle. I stuck my head out of the open door and she looked straight into my eyes, saying, almost gleefully, "It's funny that you're going through all this trouble, thinking you can keep me from doing it again. If I'm going to do it, I'll find a way. You can't take away everything."

Ignoring her comment, I finished in her closet, then went to the kitchen and did the same. All the while, I kept her beside me to make certain she didn't hurt herself again. I worked quietly, hoping to hide the whole thing from Michael and Monica. Even though I thought I was doing so up to this point, I realized I could not be open and honest about what was happening. It was still so new. I did not yet understand that secrecy and shame are enemies of the mentally ill.

Once finished with my panic-driven frenetic activity, I settled down with Chloe and we talked. In deep despair, she admitted, "Mom, I hear voices and sounds that aren't real. I've heard them for a long time. I didn't tell anybody because I didn't want you to know how crazy I am."

My interior froze. I felt blank, raw, and cold all at once. I did not want to hear this, did not want this to be. My inner voice shrieked, "Goddamn it. I do not like this. I do not want this. I will not accept this. No!"

Aloud, I very calmly asked, "How long have you heard them?"

"Since seventh grade, when I was twelve or thirteen."

Five years.

For five years, my girl had known that something was terribly wrong, yet soldiered on. Until that moment, the gravity of her illness had eluded me. At that moment, I flashed back to the comment I'd made about not being like her grandma. I couldn't believe that words I'd used to comfort were as sharp and cutting as the razor I'd removed from her hand. Here was another lesson. Another mistake I would not repeat. But, oh, it was so painful.

We continued to talk about the reality of her illness. "What are the voices like? Do they talk directly to you?"

"No, it's not like that. It's like background noise. Like I'm in a huge room and everybody's talking in loud whispers and different languages. Sometimes I hear a word or a phrase that I recognize, but mostly it's whisperings that I can't understand."

"Like the tower of Babel."

"Yeah, I guess it is like that."

"Does it happen all the time, or at certain times?"

"Sometimes it seems like it's only there at night or when I'm alone. Then sometimes I think it's there all the time, and I only notice when it's quiet outside of me. That's why I always want music or the TV on. I'm afraid of the quiet because then I'll hear the voices."

"So they don't tell you to do things?"

"No. Not really. Well, I don't know."

"What do you mean?"

"Sometimes, it's not really a voice telling me, but more like a feeling or a pressure to do something."

"What do you feel compelled to do?"

"It wants me to throw myself through a glass door or a window. I'm afraid of glass doors and windows now because I have to force myself not to go right through them, or at least punch my arm through. When I'm thinking about a door or a window, I see pictures in my head of all the blood. I see what it would look like if I did it. I see the cuts, the bleeding, and the pieces of glass in my flesh. I have to work hard not to do it. I don't want to do it. I know it's bad and I don't want to be bad, but it's really hard not to do it."

I couldn't believe what I was hearing. How had Chloe functioned so well, for so long, despite this intense inner turmoil? No wonder her hands shook. No wonder she cried for no apparent reason. No wonder.

She is a wonder.

Chloe finally dozed off and, since sleep was utterly out of the question, I waited up for Mark. I had decided not to call him home from his game when I was sure I could manage Chloe's care on my own. He deserved what was left of his night out, since our life was obviously heading toward more challenging terrain. I also think that maybe I saw Chloe's care as something for which I was solely, or at least primarily, responsible. When I left the workforce I felt like taking care of the children had become my job, and now it seemed to me as if I'd not done my job as well as I should have.

When Mark got home I related the story, and then the two of us spent a sleepless night clutching each other in bed, listening for sounds of unrest, waiting for another bloody scene to unfold. We stood guard, sentinels against violent enemies. We had no fear of what lay beyond the walls of our home. We were engaged in a battle against demons within. We hugged, we cried, but did not talk much. Words powerful enough to express our ragged emotions did not exist.

9
Holiday Season 1999-2000

"Chaos is the name for any order that produces confusion in our minds."
— George Santayana

"...my voice fails me; my inclination indeed carries me no farther — all is confusion beyond it."
— Edmund Burke

The next day in Dr. Kahil's office, Chloe told us she couldn't distinguish between what she actually experienced, her dreams, her thoughts, things she'd read, and things she'd seen on television. I told him about the auditory and visual hallucinations she had admitted to the night before and prepared myself for what I thought would be a change in diagnosis, one even more devastating than Bipolar Disorder Having done a little research, but not yet enough, I mistakenly thought that hallucinations were exclusively symptomatic of Schizophrenia.

Patiently, Dr. Kahil told me that my assumption was common, but wrong. Then he assured us that Chloe's experiences were indeed symptomatic of Bipolar Disorder and could be managed.

"Even though your illness is more severe than I'd originally hoped, Chloe, we can manage it. I know it's hard for you to believe this right now, but you'll feel like yourself again when the medications work the way they should."

Toward this end, the doctor increased the mood-stabilizer and added an anti-psychotic to control the hallucinations and nightmares. He wanted to continue seeing Chloe every week until she stabilized and told us to call in between if something couldn't wait. His calm, matter-of-fact approach comforted us, and when we left his office, I felt a little bit better.

A few days later, we expected Mark's oldest brother and wife for a short visit. We did not cancel that plan. I wanted to talk to them about Mark's mom. She passed away a few years earlier and we'd never discussed her mental illness.

After researching both Schizophrenia and Bipolar Disorder, I knew that while not impossible, it was unusual for the two diagnoses to exist in the same family. It was far more likely that Mark's mom, Elizabeth, and Chloe suffered from the same illness. I wanted to discover everything I could about Mom's life and health before I met her when she was about sixty. I thought since Mark's brother, James, was her oldest child and twenty years Mark's senior, he would be my best source of information.

I also thought that knowing more about Mom's diagnosis and treatment history might save time in the quest to stabilize Chloe. I pinned a ridiculous amount of hope on the possibility that James and his wife Janet could shed some light on our situation.

As if unable to share our truth with anybody else, at first we pretended nothing was wrong and tried to enjoy James and Janet's company. We played cards, watched football, and caught up on family news. In some ways, we found comfort pretending everything was right as rain. It was like watching a television show about someone else.

We did not acknowledge the serious reality of Chloe's declining health and the effects it had on our family, even though her appearance and behaviors must certainly have tipped them off. We were acting out parts in a story of the ideal family where nothing goes wrong, and everything proceeds according to plan. Except that we were not, it was not, and we could not hide those truths.

On the second morning of their visit, Janet pulled me aside. "Kate, James, and I were up late last night, trying to figure out what was happening here and what to say to you."

Obviously, our inability to discuss Chloe's diagnosis openly did nothing to hide the fact that something was terribly wrong. Since Janet and I had always talked easily, I wasn't surprised when she approached me. More significantly, I knew that James, like his father and brothers, was extremely private and dubious about bringing up personal matters.

"James is so worried about Mark. He's never seen him like this. He's not at all himself. As long as I've known him, Mark's been a ball of fire, and now, it's like the flame's gone out."

It was true. Mark, always playful and optimistic, hardly smiled and rarely laughed — sure signs that trouble was afoot.

I told Janet everything.

"Oh my goodness, Kate. Why didn't you call us and tell us not to come? This is too much. We shouldn't be here."

"No, Janet. I need you here. We need to know everything you and James can tell us about Mom and her illness. I'm sure it's the same illness and it would help if you could describe her symptoms and treatment. You and James know a lot more because Mark was so little when it started."

I was desperate for guidance as we charted the course ahead, but quickly learned that the information I sought seemed not to exist.

"Oh, Kate, we can't help you. In all these years, Dad never explained Mom's illness. I'm not sure he even knows her diagnosis."

Knowing how Dad handled things over the years, Janet and James assumed that either he never sought a label for Mom's malady, or didn't understand the medical jargon surrounding her care. Much to my disappointment, I discovered that because Mark had lived with or nearer to his mom during the years her illness was most severe, he and I actually knew more about her condition, treatment, medications, and hospitalizations than they did.

Janet did tell me about letters they had received from both parents over the years, and based on those, they assumed, as I had, that she suffered from Schizophrenia, but they had never heard anything definite. In light of Chloe's recent revelations, everything we would experience the past several months, and the reams of material I would read on the subject, we agreed that Mom had been, in all likelihood, Bipolar, too.

The next day, James and Janet cut short their visit to give our family the privacy they thought we needed. In all honesty, I think James found it unbearable to see Mark in such despair, and it was too hard for them to look at Chloe, knowing how dramatically her life and her future had changed.

I understood the temptation to flee the scene.

When I felt the lowest about Chloe's health and future, I fantasized about the kind of life I wanted for her and for us. I played with ideas of miracle cures and misdiagnosis. I imagined one of her doctors suddenly saying, "Oh, we've made a mistake. Chloe isn't mentally ill, she just has a hormone imbalance...or a thyroid disorder...or..." anything but this.

Other times I imagined myself beyond her illness's influence, as if she could manage this thing on her own. I wondered, although never seriously, what she'd do, how she'd live, if we just ignored what we knew and let her go about her business. From my readings, I knew that this is exactly what thousands of parents did when they learned that their children were mentally ill. Out of desperation, exasperation, fear, or hopelessness, they abandoned the children they loved to the illness that stole them away. This partly explains why a large percentage of America's homeless youth (an estimated fifty-five to eighty-five percent, depending on the source of information) are mentally ill children — sick children, not bad children — doing the best they can, in an altered reality, with few resources, and even less hope.

Despite knowing that I would never abandon Chloe to her illness, to her demise, at times I wanted freedom. I wanted to leave, just for a little while, and take a break from the constancy of her symptoms and neediness, and my own sense of failure and inadequacy. Like during my childhood, when I yearned for a father who was not drunk and angry all the time, I longed for a new reality. I wanted to escape, but knew in my heart that true escape meant meeting this illness head on.

10
The New Year: 2000

"I see, just see skyward, great cloud masses,
Mournfully slowly they roll, silently swelling and mixing,
With at times a half-dimm'd sadden'd far-off star,
Appearing and disappearing."
  —Walt Whitman

Early in the month, I wrote in my journal: "It's clear that even with medication, therapy, confidence, and support, this illness will dictate Chloe's every day. We continually look, wonder, assess, and question, if not aloud, then in our hearts and minds. It's easy to intellectually accept and deal with the facts, but my emotional self is perpetually roiling. I'm still so sad, and anxious, and distracted. I can't focus on other things. Bipolar Disorder pervades my thoughts, invades my every hour. I want to adjust, store it away, and move forward, but it pulls me back into its furious eddy. If I feel this way, imagine how Chloe feels."

One night after Chloe went to her room, Monica came to me. Frightened and confused, she wondered aloud, "Mommy, will Chloe ever get better?" Then, "Do you think I'll have Bipolar Disorder, too?" Here it was. She finally asked, and now we could talk about it. She shared, at length, her fears and anxieties, and I tried to convey the facts about Bipolar Disorder. I didn't want to assume anything, and I didn't want to avoid the truth. I had to be open and honest.

Several years earlier, when she was eight, Monica had a bout of unexplained childhood depression. At the time, she was unable to sleep or eat, felt tearful all the time, and worried excessively. We stopped watching the evening news because she got so upset, not understanding "how people could do those things." The depression came on suddenly, out of nowhere. We were baffled and not a little distraught as we worked with a therapist to help her. It took almost six months for her to feel like herself and she didn't want to experience anything along those lines again.

Of course, we now know that this could have been an early warning of her susceptibility to Bipolar Disorder. We needed to be mindful of her mental health and act immediately if anything seemed remiss. This marked the beginning of an on going "mental-health watch" that involved critical analysis of moods and attitudes, and careful consideration of what might and might not be normal. Monica was not the only one watching, and analyzing, and wondering about norms.

Michael had seen and heard a lot lately, and Chloe had shared a few of her experiences with him during the past several months. It was beginning to wear on him, and he, who had always been attuned to his and other's feelings, was even more sensitive than usual. He did not want to talk about what was going on, but showed signs of perpetual worry. He used to bring friends home daily, but now only occasionally. He began hanging out at other people's houses to avoid Chloe's irritability and the inevitable arguments when she said things he considered irrational or selfish.

Other things about Michael also changed. Although his old friends were still in the picture, new names came up in conversation, many of them people Mark and I would never meet. Years later Michael told us that these were "bad kids" and he didn't want them around us then, didn't want us to know about them. But I didn't see this at the time. I saw a young man, no longer happy or well, and attributed the change to the stress of living with a seriously mentally ill sibling.

Any chronic illness affects not only the sick child, but everyone else in the family, too. At this point, I'd not developed my own centeredness, my own ability to live in the now. How could I imbue those traits in my children and others with the confidence to move forward despite great odds? I was a neophyte at this advanced level of spiritual development. It would be months, maybe years, before I felt comfort and hope in all that I had and all that I, we, could be. In the meantime, we struggled. Our son became as enmeshed in this snare as his sister.

Michael looked tired all the time, sporting dark circles under his eyes that proved sleep was no longer regular or restful. He often slept with his light on and got up frequently during the night to check on Chloe. When I asked about it, he would reply, "I don't want to talk about it. I don't want to know about it. It's just weird. Chloe is just weird. It makes me mad."

His feelings were as vague as they sounded. He didn't know if he was mad at Chloe or mad at her illness, but he was definitely mad. He was frightened of having Bipolar Disorder himself, but didn't share that for a very long time. At a loss, Mark and I tried not to push and hoped Michael would gain insight and understanding, and that he'd develop empathy not only for Chloe, but also for others whose lives took unexpected turns.

On a more positive note, Chloe began talking more about her illness and medical treatment. The side effects of the medications, the length of time it took to dose them properly, and most of all, the fact that she had to take them, frustrated her. She even wondered if it was right to take any meds since "the doctors really don't know what they're doing and I'm just a guinea pig. Maybe what they're prescribing right now will cause more harm than good."

She opened up one day, sharing some serious thoughts: "I wonder if I should just tell Dr. Kahil to put me in the hospital. If I were in the hospital, the staff could monitor my meds and their side effects. They could see how I behave and react. I could tell them how I feel every day. Then they could adjust dosages more quickly, and it would take less time to get the mix right."

More significantly, though, she shared her fears about treatment, fears that are common in mentally ill patients, fears that keep many people from seeking treatment: "There's no way I want to be like everybody else. I've always been different, smarter even. It seems like the goal is to take away my uniqueness, the things that make me exceptional. The meds tranquilize my creativity and extinguish my best qualities. I'm not sure I want to do this. Does making me well mean making me like everybody else? Making me average? I've never been average and I don't ever want to be."

"Oh, Chloe," I assured her, "you will never be average."

I felt sadness and disappointment at having to have these conversations. Never in my wildest dreams did I imagine this sort of trial. I was coming to understand that we enter this life to learn, and moving through challenging times with grace and dignity allows us to develop strength, wisdom, and compassion. I was beginning to understand that this trial was a training ground. By virtue of Chloe's illness, we could grow, be better people, and become stronger souls.

I was learning to do that. When I taught in public schools I frequently developed opinions about why "challenging children" behaved poorly. More often than not, I blamed their parents. I held the self-righteous notion that I worked hard to raise happy, well-rounded children and that if other parents took their responsibilities seriously and parented effectively, their children would be fine. Boy was I getting mine. Living with a mentally ill teen, spending lots of time in the psychiatrist's waiting room, and thoroughly researching the topic chipped away at my arrogance and ignorance. I began to change.

My journal addresses facets of this growth: "I am increasingly aware of the inaccuracy and uselessness of judging others. So much takes place beyond our perception, our sphere of knowledge. We never know a full story or understand the complete scenario. Unfettering from the destructive habit of judging others is liberating. I realize, too, that this liberation is a direct result of being broken, humbled. It's an effect of going through great challenge and emerging a changed person. It's the product of 'the refiner's fire.' My personal impurities are burning away. I'm being bettered rather than bested."

11

Early January 2000

"The art of life is a constant readjustment to our surroundings."
—Kakuzo Okakaura

The first day of the second semester, I waited in the high school counselor's office to discuss a schedule change. Chloe felt worse than during the previous term, and I was determined to ease some of the pressure so she could concentrate on healing. Although she had to take one more semester of government and senior English, she'd already earned six credits beyond what was required for graduation. I thought it fair to reduce her course load to the two required classes. According to district policy, however, she had to enroll in at least three courses and her high school administration had its own policy requiring seniors to take four or more classes in order to participate in graduation exercises. I spent the better part of two days collecting letters of explanation and recommendation from Dr. Sander, Dr. Kahil, and Maria, and discussing options with her teachers, the counseling staff, and administrators.

Having worked with Chloe the preceding semester and learning of her worsening health, her government teacher requested her as his teacher's aide for the hour between which she took his course and English. This arrangement fulfilled the district requirement of enrollment in three classes. Even with that suggestion and letters verifying the medical need for a reduced class load, the vice-principal decided not to "disregard school policy" and insisted that Chloe be on campus four periods a day.

I'd had it. Sparing no detail, I graphically described what Chloe had been through. I ended my discourse telling this man that Chloe would end up in the hospital at best, dead at worst, if he couldn't see the gravity of the situation and bend his rules in the interest of her well-being. He would not. I asked to speak to the principal.

Fortunately, she got it. Minutes after presenting the information I'd collected during the previous two days, I left the school with Chloe's schedule in hand—no first or second periods so she could sleep, 3rd hour Government, 4th hour teacher's aide, 5th hour Senior English, end of day. Another battle fought and won. Thank goodness.

Despite our success, I could not help wondering about other students in Chloe's situation whose parents were either unable or unwilling to push for what was right. They were doomed to unnecessary hardship, even failure, by the system. I grieved for the number of young people whose only offense was illness, whose lives would always be difficult or dangerous. Nonetheless, I felt relief by gaining the school's cooperation. In a few days, I was doubly relieved to deal with only two courses when it became obvious that Chloe's medications were doing a number on her brain.

Since her suicide attempt and because it was winter, Chloe wore only long sleeves. I knew she wanted to hide the scar on her wrist from her brother and sister, and everyone else for that matter. She was embarrassed and did not want visible signs of her failed attempt. I am not sure whether she was ashamed of having tried or ashamed of having failed, but she wanted no discussion, no reference, to the incident.

Because it was such a frightening event for me, I relentlessly watched for indications that she was in danger of hurting herself again. My perpetual attention had to be irritating. My values knotted as I tried to prioritize my responsibilities. I was frightened, untrusting, and nosy. I invaded her privacy in the name of keeping her safe.

On one of these occasions I walked into the room before she was dressed and saw what looked like razor marks up and down the inside of both arms. Grabbing her hands and turning them to get a better view, I jumped into a diatribe.

"Chloe. What are you trying to do? Are you determined to kill yourself? What are you cutting with?" (I thought I had removed all access to razors.) "Why didn't you come to me? You promised you'd talk to me if you felt like hurting yourself. Why are you doing this?" WHY?"

Unanswered questions raced through my mind and out of my mouth. When I finally gave her a moment to speak, she did.

"I'm not trying to kill myself. I will tell you if I feel that way again. I'm just cutting, and I don't know why. It feels good to feel the pain. It lets out all the stuff that's building up inside me. I feel like I'll totally lose control if I don't relieve the pressure."

She went on to explain that she felt compelled to cut, and that cutting her own flesh with a safety pin or a straight pin, seeing her blood run, provided relief. The pain temporarily removed her from the greater pain of her illness, which was unrelenting, unbearable.

I searched the Internet and my growing personal library on mental illness to learn more about self-injurious behavior. I found that it's common among teens with emotional or mental illness, and that it is a medical issue, not a discipline problem. I discovered that thousands of young people, more girls than boys, habitually cut themselves for the very reasons Chloe described. It briefly distracts them from personal, perpetual pain.

In *The Bipolar Child, The Definitive and Reassuring Guide to Childhood's Most Misunderstood Disorder*, authors Demitri and Janice Papolos say, "One theory about...self-mutilating behaviors is that a powerful impulse to discharge aggression is counterpoised against the individual's attempt to inhibit that impulse. The tension created by these conflicting forces builds to an unbearable pitch, and the tension is relieved by physical pain directed toward self. This discharge of aggression and the concomitant activation of the pain pathways could act as a cathartic release, but no one really understands what exactly is happening and why hurting one's self resolves the problem temporarily."

Like many habits, self-mutilation tends to increase in frequency and severity, making early detection and elimination important. I realized there should be no shame or punishment in response to the cutting, but Chloe needed to know that it had stop.

During our weekly appointment with Dr. Kahil, Chloe and I once again enumerated the existing symptoms of her illness, including deep depression, frequent anxiety and panic attacks, difficulty sleeping, gruesome dreams, continued weight gain, severe hair loss, and now, cutting. Usually low-key, Dr. Kahil swiftly and sternly told Chloe that cutting was not an acceptable behavior. He asked her to talk to Maria about it and to develop alternative behaviors for when she felt compelled to cut. He wanted her word that she would make every effort to stop this unhealthy habit. He also changed her medications since she was not improving and the side effects were so bad, she was threatening to stop taking them anyway. Then Chloe began taking Lithium.

Lithium was one of the first drugs to show significant promise in treating Bipolar Disorder, and is widely used today. In a February 2000 paper entitled "Does Lithium Still Work?" authors R J Baldessarini and L. Tondo reviewed eleven controlled and thirteen open long-term Lithium treatment trials for Bipolar or mixed major affective disorders that were conducted between 1970 and 1996. In addition to the review of studies, patients seen at a mood-disorder center were also evaluated with several established psychiatric and diagnostic assessment methods.

The compiled data indicated Lithium effectiveness in nearly seventy percent of patients. I'd wondered why it was not the first medication prescribed based on its long history of success and relative affordability. I later learned that it is not as effective for patients with a severe anxiety component or those who are rapid cycling, both of which described Chloe. However, Depakote was not the answer, so Dr. Kahil decided to try Lithium.

Lithium induced changes in Chloe's brain and body chemistry almost immediately. Within two weeks, my journal entry chronicles the most significant differences: "Chloe cannot read right now. Her eyes don't focus; they jump around on the page. Even more difficult, though, her mind seems rewired. She doesn't process information the way she always did. It's as if she's developed a learning disability. When she gets her eyes to cooperate, the printed words don't connect in a meaningful way.

She reads a phrase and it makes no sense. If I say the same phrase, she understands it. Dr. Kahil thinks these are side effects from the Lithium and should abate within a month. In the meantime, I read school assignments to her, and she tape-records each class for later review. Thank goodness she has exceptional auditory learning skills because at the moment she's relying on them exclusively."

In addition to reading *A Tale of Two Cities*, *Les Miserables*, and various government assignments, I spent additional hours reading books about Bipolar Disorder, including *Bipolar Disorder* by Fancis Mark Mondimore and *An Unquiet Mind* by Kay Redfield Jamison. Between writing my own book, going through Chloe's readings, and learning all I could about her illness, I felt like a full-time student. I learned the medical terms related to mental illness, as well as symptoms and medication side effects. I was becoming expert on many aspects of the illness because I couldn't gain control any other way. I had to learn everything I could in order to make informed decisions and anticipate potential problems.

When I decided to be Chloe's best advocate, I committed myself to being well informed. Although it took time, I'd make the same choice today. The learning process, the accumulation of facts and theories, helped me to get a grasp on the illness. For reasons difficult to explain, developing competence with medical jargon and related information empowered me. I figured if I could understand all of this, I could certainly deal with it. In fact, dealing with it led to my intellectual, emotional, and spiritual growth. Had I not involved myself so deeply, I would have missed the blessings and inner peace I now possess.

As is the case with learning, the more we know the more we realize we don't know. The Lithium treatment was fraught with problems. One of the first emerged during one of the twice-monthly blood tests to monitor Lithium levels in Chloe's blood, as well as her kidney and thyroid function. Chloe was hypothyroid, meaning she had too little of the hormone produced by the thyroid gland. Since low thyroid can, in itself, cause depression, Dr. Kahil prescribed Synthroid to augment her levels.

Irrationally hopeful, I wondered aloud if the whole problem could simply be a thyroid imbalance. My hopes evaporated as the doctor said the thyroid problem could be a small part of the picture, but in no way the cause. In fact, he said, the Lithium probably caused the thyroid imbalance since that is its most common side effect. So Chloe added another pill to the daily regime and we moved forward with work, school, and occasionally, play.

January turned to February. Chloe and I both felt doubtful and disappointed with her progress. She'd not made it through an entire week of school without missing a day or more, and was still unable to read or process written information. The extreme anxiety abated, but she was afraid to be alone, and panicked at that possibility. If I had a commitment away from home, Chloe came along, or one of the other children stayed with her. Occasionally these options were unavailable, so I'd assign household chores, like vacuuming or scouring bathtubs, to keep her physically busy and distracted. Still, she hated being alone and I hated leaving her that way, always thinking back to the day Maria called me while I was at the coffee shop with Tina.

Commitments to anything outside our immediate family no longer held much value. I needed to be home. I spent hours on the phone arranging medical care and sharing information with doctors. I spent equal time researching and learning about the illness, its treatment, medications, and side effects. In addition to Michael and Monica's sports and school activities, I drove Chloe to and from three or more medical appointments a week, and to and from school. Then there was time spent on her school-related activities. Every day was full and I began to appreciate our good fortune that I could be home.

How did families manage when their children became ill and neither parent could be fully available? How did they provide the necessary care and get to all the appointments? I'm convinced that my being home prevented lengthy hospitalizations, maybe even kept Chloe alive. We were lucky and I knew it, but the burden of responsibility felt heavy and, again, I grew weary.

Chloe was utterly miserable. Since the medications were not working, she felt at the mercy of this life-changing illness. As we faced the daily challenges together, I felt like the diagnosis was also mine. My life had changed dramatically, and like her, I abandoned long-laid plans in adjustment to our new reality. From childhood, I envisioned the perfect family and created

myriad opinions of what life should be like and what a good
mother was. After years of working toward those ideals, I found
that neither my life nor my mothering skills met my high
expectations. I was my greatest critic and my greatest
disappointment.

Like many mothers of chronically ill children, I couldn't
release the notion that I'd "done this" to Chloe. My self-talk was
peppered with "should-haves." I should have known that our
biology, our genetic backgrounds, would put my children at risk. I
should have seen the signs earlier and sought treatment sooner. I
should have parented differently. I should have done this. I should
have done that. I should have … I should have … I should have.

I grew sad, disappointed, and angry. Then, I felt profoundly
ashamed of those feelings. It took a long time to untangle the knots
of emotion and even longer to accept them. When I stopped feeling
guilty and objectively analyzed the situation, I realized my
resentment grew because I'd not taken care of myself. Here I was, a
healthy, capable woman, failing to acknowledge my limitations and
needs. This realization hit me like a ton of bricks. I, and only I, am in
charge of the way I feel. I am responsible for myself. My happiness
is my own creation, and taking care of myself is a true
responsibility, since I'm useless to others without my own sense of
well-being.

I began to plan regular, renewing activities that fit into the
tiny pockets of opportunity our routine afforded. Having always
been spiritual and deeply connected to God, I focused my
prayers on acceptance, on releasing judgment. I made daily
meditation a priority. If Chloe managed to go to school, Tina, or
another friend, Barbra, would meet me at the coffee shop on
very short notice. Sometimes I rented a video and watched it
when I found two quiet hours. I continued to read everything I
could find on Bipolar Disorder, but made a point of reading for
pleasure, too.

I spent time outdoors, working in the garden and relishing
the fresh air, and I got some exercise every day, even if it was
only a quick walk after dinner. Most significantly, I regularly
wrote in my journal, documenting Chloe's illness and progress,
our family's reactions, and venting my emotions. This writing
practice was particularly therapeutic, helping me to learn

acceptance without judgment, to seek solutions without placing blame, and to recognize and appreciate our blessings.

When families live with and learn about a loved one's illness, each member gains experience and knowledge that ultimately benefits. Repeatedly my family and I discover deep and profound lessons we would not have learned under different circumstances.

One of our biggest lessons came when Chloe and I described her affect and moods to Dr. Kahil. Because we were individuals with unique filters, experiences, and memory processes, we perceived and related the same situations quite differently. After many weeks of noticing these differences, we began to respect and marvel at the variability of truth and reality.

I began to see divine purposes to our challenges, and grew in my ability to accept and understand their real meaning. Because of our struggles, each of us engaged more deeply in an understanding of God and spirituality. As we searched for answers, we asked more questions, sometimes of one another, sometimes of ourselves, and sometimes of God. We explored our beliefs and worked to understand true meanings. Some of us embraced God and spirituality more tightly. Some of us rejected them more adamantly. Each of us searched, grew, and changed.

Don't get me wrong...I did not like, even for one moment, the fact that my child was ill. To this day, I would not choose some of the experiences we have had. However, I know that they have fostered strength and character that would otherwise have remained elusive. I see the rightness in the plan, even if the details are sometimes terribly unwelcome.

Anther big lesson was the relativity of "normal." Many details of our daily lives fall outside the realm of what we used to consider normal. Now we know that normal is a subjective state. What is normal for one is abnormal for another. This seems so simple, but is not how most people live. Most of us function under the assumption that what we perceive as right or normal is, indeed, the norm. Such is not the case. Having learned this through experience, and the fluctuating state of our norm, we are less judgmental, less inclined to assume. We accept others more freely, tolerate differences, and understand the deceptiveness of outward appearances. We are wiser. Is not wisdom the goal? We learn so much when forced to do so.

12
January 2000

"Avoid a remedy that is worse than the disease."
— Aesop

The Lithium experiment was short lived. In just a few weeks, Chloe suffered nearly every negative side effect attributed to this wonder drug. It suppressed her thyroid function, brought on additional weight gain, aggravated her acne, and caused loss of bladder control. Even with the addition of Synthroid, her thyroid level remained too low. This could have caused the weight gain, but sometimes Lithium increases weight even when thyroid function remains uncompromised. Additionally, she retained water because her kidneys and bladder were not functioning properly. But this was not the worst of it.

One evening I went into Chloe's room and sat next to her on the floor.

"Did you see that black man?" she asked.

"No, I didn't. Where was he?"

"He was just here, he was talking to me."

"Chloe, no one was here."

"Oh, I guess he went back into my leg. That is where he came from. He floated up out of my leg."

I didn't know what to say, so said nothing as Chloe peered into my eyes. Then a look of confusion washed across her face and she said, "That couldn't really happen, could it? A man couldn't really come out of my leg."

"No, you're right, that couldn't really happen."

"Oh, Mama, I can't tell what's real and what's not."

We were back in the doctor's office the next day.

Dr. Kahil took Chloe off Lithium and slowly introduced Tegretol, the last of the three most-often used mood stabilizers. I was encouraged by this change when I learned that Tegretol was as effective in as many cases as Lithium, but that it often worked for patients who did not respond to Lithium. In particular, Tegretol seemed to be the most effective mood stabilizer for rapid-cycling patients like Chloe. We learned that Chloe fell into this more difficult to treat category when we began to document her moods. A few weeks of charting based on my observations and Chloe's self-analysis verified what we thought to be true.

Chloe sometimes cycled through numerous mood states in a single day. This was dramatic since the rapid-cycling sub-diagnosis (the most frequent sub-diagnosis for Adolescent Onset Bipolar Disorder) usually applies to patients who cycle through three or more changes over the course of a *year*. We were fighting a pattern that demanded constant observation, analysis, and treatment adjustment.

Dr. Kahil warned us that the Tegretol would take at least a month to induce change once he got the dose at a therapeutic level, and it had to be titrated (gradually increased) before we'd get to that point. It seemed like a long time to wait for improvement, but at least we had hope again.

During this period, Chloe was still unable to read or process information. Dr. Kahil now thought these side effects resulted from the antipsychotic Risperdal, but would not take her off it until she was stable. For now, keeping her alive and out of the hospital were the primary goals.

Chloe was miserable. Puffed up from weight and water gain, skin breaking out, and often unable to make it to the bathroom in time, she no longer possessed a shred of self-confidence. What the illness didn't strip away, the medications did. It took every bit of her determination to continue to work on school assignments.

More than being committed to the doctor's plan, Chloe was determined to please Mark and me. She only took her meds because I brought them to her. If I failed to do this, she ignored them. She frequently expressed doubt that the medical community could effectively treat her, and unfortunately, her experiences thus far supported that theory.

In many ways, she was as bad as, or worse, than before treatment began. She often threatened to stop taking her prescriptions, but never fought me when I gave them to her. As I read about other young people in treatment, I learned that a refusal to follow doctor's orders, often called medication noncompliance, was almost universal. However, Chloe wanted to please us. Unlike many teens with Bipolar Disorder, she did not feel suspicious of us or paranoid about our intentions, and she did not rebel against treatment. She knew that we loved and respected her, and that we were trying to help. Whatever we asked of her she did out of love, respect, and obedience. Her willingness to obey and her desire to please us were huge blessings not often enjoyed by parents in our situation. I was grateful.

Winter Formal was coming up and a group of seniors asked Chloe to join them for the evening. Her initial reaction was horror at the thought of attending a public activity in light of her weight and acne. Her friends and I convinced her that it would be fun, so she acquiesced and went shopping for a dress. What a challenge. Needing a larger than normal size, she felt depressed and discouraged as she tried on dress after dress, feeling unattractive in each one. I wanted to turn this into a positive experience, not another disappointment. I suggested she look at styles, not sizes. If she saw one she liked, I pulled two or three sizes and she tried them for the best fit. It worked. In a short time, she found a dress.

After finding what she needed in the lingerie department, we headed to the cosmetics counter where Chloe and a clerk experimented until they discovered a product that offered natural-looking coverage. We picked it up along with eye shadows and blush that Chloe was excited to try. She seemed happy for the first time in months. A quick lunch out and we drove home, ebullient by our success. A feeling of normalcy, absent from our lives for quite some time, permeated that afternoon. It was a gift. We enjoyed one another's company, sharing smiles and happy conversation. That day became a fond memory folded into a series of others that highlight our remarkable relationship. I have learned to appreciate every little thing, because sometimes little things are as good as it gets.

Chloe went to that dance and had fun, too. We have the photos to prove it. Her friends were wonderful, getting ready at our house, doing their hair, and asking Chloe to do their makeup. She felt appreciated and a part of things after being out of the loop for so long. I was grateful for the girls' ability to support her in the best possible ways. This would not always be the case, but for that evening, Chloe was an average seventeen-year-old. We were happy when she walked out the door and equally happy when she safely returned. We learned to embrace one of the hallmarks of Bipolar Disorder—the occurrence of seemingly normal behaviors embedded within periods of great disarray. I thanked God that the timing was so right, and she felt well enough to enjoy herself.

The dance left Chloe exhausted, verifying the great effort it took for her to function normally. I gained great respect for her strong will after this event, and understood that fragility was the constant companion of her incredible determination. She spent the next couple of weeks catching up as she struggled to go to school, listen to lectures again at home, and read her assignments with me. She felt tired all the time, and was irritable. Since I was with her more than anyone else was, I caught a fair amount of verbal abuse. As enlightened as I wanted to be, I still lost my cool and my patience.

13
Late January 2000

"God wants to see more love and playfulness in your eyes, for that is your greatest witness to him."
— Hafiz

Still a bit selfish, I couldn't accept some aspects of our reality, and rebelled when I would have benefited from trying to gain understanding. I spent most of my time caring for Chloe and it ticked me off when she was oblivious to that fact and took out her frustration on me. I gritted my teeth and "suffered in silence," becoming a martyr as I allowed her to lash out. After a while, I lost patience and grew equally snappy with her. Once I allowed myself that outlet, it grew, and I became snappy with the rest of my family too. Then they grew snappy with me. What a fiasco. In no time, we were in caught in an eddy of uproar, our family a swirling ball of tension.

The joy and contentment that I thought was ours grew elusive and tears of sadness and anger were the norm. Since a family's moods and interactions often follow the tone set by the matriarch, I knew that if I wanted harmony to return to our home, the change had to begin with me. I had to cultivate an attitude of acceptance, a determination to respect and articulate my own needs and boundaries, and mostly, greater patience.

The journey that Chloe and I shared was as beneficial as it was difficult. I became less selfish and adopted a nonjudgmental attitude toward her behaviors. I told her when her words and actions were hurtful, but didn't overreact with emotion. After all, nothing anybody else says can change the person I am. I choose who I am. I grew determined to be happy. I decided to live with Bipolar Disorder in a loving way. I realized that in the end, it was all about love any way. Of course, this was, and is, a process, and sometimes I'm less "together" than others, but during this period I made great personal gains. I honed my ability to discern between the significant and the insignificant, and to recognize what was mine to correct and what was best ignored.

I also, unconsciously, reorganized my belief system. As long as I can remember, I'd sought greater understanding of the spiritual, even religious, realm. I spent early childhood Sunday mornings with my grandparents at their Nazarene church, and later caught the bus that rolled past my childhood home and carried me to a terrific little Church of Christ. In high school, I attended a Baptist church with one friend and Catholic mass with another, and I graduated from a small, Brethren college. I also studied other religions, including Buddhism, Hinduism, and Islam. Our family also spent eight years attending the Church of Jesus Christ of Latter Day Saints and actively practicing the Mormon faith.

I had a thorough background in the various avenues men choose to approach God and godliness. Despite the years of study and unusually intense interest, nothing transformed me the way I transformed then. I instinctively knew that I could be the person I wanted to be only by releasing judgment, embracing acceptance, and fully living in the moment. I grew in strength and wisdom.

14
Early February 2000

"The love, clarity and compassion that emerge within the individual that chooses consciously to align itself with its soul is the same that will bring sexes, races, nations and neighbors into harmony with each other."
— Gary Zukav

One morning a phone call from the middle school principal tested my newly gained strength. Michael had been in a fight and received a two-day suspension as punishment. When I picked him up from school, I heard the whole story. After several days of verbal repartee, the two boys entered into a shoving match punctuated by a thrown punch, which Michael handily dodged. After knocking down the other boy, Michael pummeled him, breaking his own hand in the process.

The vice principal submitted that the other boy was the instigator and thus received an additional day's suspension, but I was aghast that Michael had resorted to this degree of violence. In the end, he missed more school than the other student because threats levied against him left administrators unable to guarantee his safety. For several additional days, I picked him up from school early to avoid interaction with the other boy and his friends.

As we talked about the causes and consequences of his behavior, Michael admitted he felt terribly anxious. Things that normally didn't bother him made him angry.

"I feel edgy and anxious all the time, like I'm always on the verge of something. I'm frustrated and scared, but I don't know why."

These were new sensations for Michael. I attributed them not only to his age, but also to the stress of dealing with Chloe's illness and the accompanying changes in our home and family life over the past several months. Reflecting on those changes, I realized how oddly our routine had evolved.

Monday through Friday, Monica and Michael went to school and sports, as they always had. Mark went to work and I took care of the house, garden, and Chloe. Once everyone was home again, very little was the same. We modulated our voices, television volumes, and music levels to meet Chloe's needs. We ate dinner together as we always had, but Chloe often returned to the couch or her bed rather quickly. As we ate, we talked about everyone's day, and shared the neighborhood news. This was the only conversation time not revolving around Bipolar Disorder, prescriptions, side effects, or medical appointments. The topic invaded every facet of our lives.

Both Monica and Michael resented the changes. Impulsive and grandiose, both symptomatic of her illness, Chloe borrowed things without asking and went in their rooms without knocking. Common courtesies no longer mattered to her. Taking care of her took most of my time, leaving little one-on-one with Michael and Monica. They felt ignored, lost in the shuffle. They grew increasingly intolerant of her moods and complained that she always "got her way." They were right. I should not have been surprised that Michael's pent-up emotions erupted at school. We lived our lives around an illness. I failed to appreciate the serious effects of Bipolar Disorder on our family.

Mark and I talked at length, trying to figure out how to give Chloe the care and attention she required while providing a normal, balanced home life. I sought information about a local mental-health support group only to discover that none existed in our community. It was back to books and the Internet, searching for information on the effects of chronic childhood and adolescent illnesses on family units and other children in the home.

I learned more than I wanted to know, and admit now that I ignored obvious indicators of additional trouble in an unconscious act of self-preservation. It was a long time before I could look at the entire picture and honestly identify the facts, particularly where Michael was concerned. I refused to believe this would happen to two of our children.

15
February 2000

"And this too shall pass away. How much it expresses! How chastening in the hour of pride! How consoling in the depths of affliction!"
— Abraham Lincoln

The day after Michael's fight and suspension, he and I spent hours at the orthopedist getting his hand x-rayed, set, and then cast in gauze and plaster. The doctor was familiar with the injury and knew exactly how Michael sustained it. He called it a "boxer's fracture," and spoke candidly with Michael about anger management and self-control. He placed significant emphasis on, and seemed more than a little concerned by, Michael's age.

Michael was only fourteen and, according to the doctor, these injuries usually occurred in young men between the ages of seventeen and twenty-five and most often, he said, in college students who'd had too much to drink. Although I listened intently, I rationalized that the last few months had challenged us all, and while Michael's reactions were neither sound nor healthy, they were explainable, if not understandable. His injury was an outward sign of the war waging within our family. Knowing that this doctor was a temporary player in our big game of life, I didn't even try to engage him in a discussion of what was really going on. On the other hand, maybe I didn't want to hear what he might say.

After a long day in the medical trenches, that night we fought another skirmish in the Bipolar battle. Home alone while I was with Michael, Chloe's anxiety built. By early evening, the sensations swelled, ultimately ballooning into a full-blown anxiety attack. Curled into fetal position, her jaw clenched so tightly she had difficulty speaking, her head and hands shook furiously. She thrashed at her face, neck, and chest, leaving small scratches and red marks. Unable to reach Dr. Kahil, I spoke with the psychiatrist on call. She advised me to give Chloe Ativan. Remembering her reaction to Ativan in the emergency room, I hesitated and expressed my concerns. Together, the doctor and I decided to try half an Ativan and wait an hour. If she did not improve or refused to take it, I would admit her to the hospital. It seemed like a sound plan.

After trying for nearly an hour to elicit Chloe's cooperation, I gave up in frustration and called Mark away from a business dinner. I would need his help to get her to the hospital, but thought he might be able to convince her to take the medication and avoid that scenario. Home within thirty minutes, he joined me in cajoling and threatening Chloe in an effort to keep her at home.

Fortunately, the two of us persuaded her to take the pill rather than go to the hospital. In less than an hour she relaxed, falling asleep on a blanket next to my bed soon after. The massive amounts of adrenaline her body produced in extreme anxiety, combined with the Ativan, left her deeply fatigued for days. We called Dr. Kahil. We changed meds again.

The change in medication seemed to abate the crisis and my attention turned back to Michael. A muscular, robust young man, he had lots of energy and an ever-present, infectious smile. He played soccer and football, volunteered in the community during the summer, and excelled in school. Until the recent fight at school, he had had no real conflicts with friends or classmates. However, a few weeks after his suspension for fighting, his routine took a radical turn.

Running a fever and complaining of a sore throat and headache, Michael stayed home from school and I took him to the doctor. Since he'd been unusually tired and lacked an appetite, the doctor tested him for mononucleosis. He had it, and the severity caused swollen glands and a badly enlarged spleen. Because even minor trauma to the abdomen could rupture his spleen, and the fatigue of rigorous training would weaken him, Dr. Sander forbade sports for a year. This was a terrible blow.

When he was four or five years old, we went to the local high school games and cheered for family friends. Michael loved the camaraderie and spent the intervening years talking about playing football and soccer when he was in high school. Now he had to sit out his sophomore year, and feared he'd fall permanently behind after that extended time off. Depression ensued.

Because of the severity of the mono, Michael spent the second semester of that year on a modified schedule that allowed him to sleep an extra hour and avoid the physical stress of P.E. By late afternoon, he needed to sleep and had a hard time doing all of his homework. Because he'd always had low blood sugar and had learned to manage his diet fairly well, he ate to avoid feeling shaky and headachy, but never felt hungry. He still spent time with friends on weekends, regretting it when exhaustion set in on Sunday or Monday. It took months for him to recover and regain his strength. During that time, Chloe avoided crisis, but was not well.

Throughout the spring, we spent a lot of time at the lab. Regular blood tests helped Dr. Sander monitor Michael's improvement and Dr. Kahil to manage Chloe's medication blood levels and check her liver and kidney functions. Michael did fine, but Chloe's veins became uncooperative. Sometimes it took three or four failed sticks before the nurse was able to get blood. We finally learned which nurse was most adept, and requested only her. Sometimes we waited longer, but got through faster than if we'd gone through the multi-stick process. Warm, friendly relationships with the healthcare workers that often saw my children made the process much easier. I appreciated their helpful, professional concern.

Michael slowly felt better, but his spleen remained dangerously enlarged. His plan to convince the doctor to lift the yearlong ban on contact sports fell apart when physical exams verified that his spleen was still inflamed. Even though Dr. Sander explained that a blow to the abdomen would likely rupture his spleen and cause him to bleed to death before he could get to a hospital for medical care, he resented her for refusing to sign a medical release. In addition, he resented me for going along with her and refusing to take him to another doctor who "knew what she was doing." He lamented that he would "never catch up," never be able, after a year off, to improve his skills and bulk up enough to compete. His anger overshadowed the depth of his depression.

Chloe, too, struggled. The new medication not only aggravated her acne, but also made her hair fall out. She put her foot down during one of our weekly visits to Dr. Kahil's office. "I'm not only fat and broken out, but now I'm going bald. There is no way I'll keep taking Depakote. I'd rather die than live this way." She meant it.

Mark and I understood Chloe's distress. Her appearance had radically changed, and we, too, felt sad and discouraged when her bloated physique refused to return to its once-thin form, her skin reverted to its worst state, and her lustrous hair became dry, brittle, and thin. Despite sympathizing with her physical state, we were more worried about her deteriorating emotional well-being. Even though we continually assured her that the side effects were temporary, we questioned her ability to withstand much more. We were on suicide watch again, suspicious of every unusual action or comment. Dr. Kahil reminded me of hospitalization procedures and, again, initiated yet another medication change.

16
Late February/March 2000

"Just trust yourself, and then you will know how to live."
—Goethe

From my journal on 14 February 2000: "I'm sad. I want to cry, scream, run away. I've lost the life I always thought I'd have. Michael is silent and surly, angry because he can't play sports, Chloe's not making much progress, and I need a break. There's no time for a break because their needs are so great. I have a marriage, family, home and garden, and a publisher's deadline. I'm a week late getting to a client's, and Mark and I haven't had "alone time" in weeks. I love date nights and they're gone. We didn't even go out on our anniversary, too exhausted from the week's challenges, and Chloe wasn't stable enough to be home without us for the evening.

"I read *A Brilliant Madness* by Patty Duke this weekend and feel discouraged, almost jealous, because she responded to Lithium and Chloe did not. I know Chloe's illness is the rapid-cycling type. I know it's difficult to treat and control. Will I be her caregiver for the rest of my life? I love her. She's brilliant and has so much potential if this illness can be controlled, but I fear she'll never fulfill plans and dreams. The disappointment! I've expected too much."

From my journal on 15 February 2000: "It's a better day...I'm less sad. I benefited from writing my thoughts and feelings yesterday, clearing and examining them, then moving on. I achieved a lot in the last twenty-four hours. It's as if a dam broke and all my capabilities surged forth. Chloe didn't go to school today. She hasn't made it every day in a given week since before Thanksgiving. Progress is slow. I realized I'd stopped exercising, so Mark and I took a long walk after dinner last night. What a difference that made. When I get moving and focus on my breath, I release tension, anxiety, and expectations. I live in the present without projecting too much discouragement into the future. Thankfully, I'm more patient, more tolerant, and more capable of dealing with everything today. I have to remember to move and breathe."

From my journal on February 17, 2000: "Chloe went to school. YAY. She couldn't manage on Tuesday. We finished reading *A Tale of Two Cities*, and she must now take a three-hour exam on the material. We begin *Hamlet* on Monday. Her processing is improving, so I'm getting my own copy to read aloud while she follows along in hers.

"Chloe decided she didn't want to see Maria any more. I made an appointment and we saw Jamie Conklin, a new therapist, yesterday. What a fruitless meeting. Chloe was antagonistic and the session resulted in nothing positive. We see Dr. Kahil this evening. I assume he'll change or increase her medication."

From my journal on February 28, 2000: "Since last week I haven't had the gumption to sit down and write. I hit an emotional wall at a high rate of speed. My "self" splattered, oozed down, and puddled at my feet.

"The past few months have drained and disappointed. Michael pulls further and further away. Chloe's progress — and mine — is one-step forward, two steps back. It's slow, erratic, and terribly frustrating. I so often think I've finally learned an eternal lesson, and then I fall back into old patterns of thinking and behaving.

"The last two weeks have been particularly discouraging. Chloe had several severe anxiety attacks, each time ending up in fetal position with fists clenched and teeth grinding. I've learned to talk her through it, coaching her to relax and visualize. We also rely heavily on anti-anxiety medication, which knocks her out and renders her non-functional for a couple of days.

One of the episodes took place in Jamie Conklin's office. Jamie ran into the waiting room to get me, nearly as anxious and agitated as Chloe. After that incident, she told me to tuck the possibility of Schizophrenia (not this again) in the back of my mind. This did not look like an anxiety attack to her. She thinks this may be the initial stage of that disease. SHIT. SHIT. SHIT.

"That's the last thing I want to hear and it makes me unreasonably angry to consider it. Somehow, I rationalize that Bipolar Disorder is not as bad as Schizophrenia. I know that, treated, Bipolar Disorder is manageable. I also know that Schizophrenia usually progresses despite treatment and ultimately destroys its victims' minds. How hard that illness is on family and friends. I don't want to do it. I do not want my precious daughter to have that. I feel like a defiant child, and my inner voice is screaming 'NO. NO. NO.'

"I asked Dr. Kahil if he still thought we were dealing with Bipolar Disorder and he said yes, but wants to order a neurological evaluation to discount the Schizophrenia possibility. Specific regions of the Schizophrenic brain function differently than a normal brain, and those differences show up on a CT scan. Since no similar test exists for Bipolar Disorder and the two illnesses have common symptomology, the search for Schizophrenic activity in the brain can either confirm or discount that diagnosis.

"I briefly mentioned it to Mark, and he said 'It doesn't matter what they call it, let's just treat it, and support her so she can get well.' I wish I could be that pragmatic, but it's a challenge. I understand the prognoses of the two illnesses. I'm aware of treatment and recovery potentials. I'm familiar with the medical perspectives and can't blindly go forth, pretending not to know these things.

"I haven't mentioned Jamie's concerns about Schizophrenia to Chloe. Let's deal with confirmed information. 'No borrowing trouble,' as Grandma used to say. I've learned not to assume too much, nor count on too much either. It's against my Pollyanna-like nature, but I'm jaded. I want to rediscover my internal optimist. Remember to walk. Breathe deeply.

"Chloe sees Dr. Sander tomorrow, Jamie on Thursday, gets a head CT on Friday, and sees Dr. Kahil again next week. She's a bit better. The new drug mix is helping. I pray this trend continues."

From my journal on March 6, 2000: "'Serene Women are not sidetracked—Sarah Ban Breathnach.' I aim for serenity.

"Chloe had the head CT on Friday. We'll pick up the results and take them to our appointment with Dr. Kahil on Thursday.

In the meantime, she has dramatically improved. She's losing weight, her demeanor and affect are more open and positive, and she's less irritable and sensitive. Her sleeping habits are normalizing and she's more capable and responsible with schoolwork. She even spent several hours with friends on Sunday—HUGE positive step. I'm cautiously optimistic that whether this is Bipolar Disorder or Schizophrenia, it's manageable. Chloe can achieve great things."

We walked into Dr. Kahil's office carrying Chloe's CT results as if they were a package made ready for the bomb squad. That's how it felt—as if the information contained within could destroy our already vulnerable lives. I don't know why I placed so much power in the possibilities of those pictures, but I did. I'd read a lot about both illnesses and convinced myself that a Bipolar diagnosis was preferable.

Dr. Kahil still felt we were dealing with Bipolar Disorder, and no matter how irrational my perspective might be, I was thrilled it was not Schizophrenia. Chloe and I had come to terms with this diagnosis and would have difficulty accepting the other. We were relieved by the news and by Chloe's waning symptoms. We also decided that Jamie Conklin was not the therapist for Chloe, and got a couple other names to investigate. While we made phone calls and initial visits, I again sympathized with families whose resources were more limited than ours or who had no access to professional guidance and support. The processes involved in receiving appropriate mental health care are difficult to navigate. We were fortunate that I had time to help Chloe, and that Mark's employer provided great medical benefits.

We were hopeful again. Things were looking up.

17
Late March 2000

"Perseverance is not a long race; it is many short races one after another."
 — Walter Elliott

For two weeks, Chloe steadily improved. She got up in the morning, went to school, completed homework with relative independence, and spent some time with friends. Although she still lacked self-confidence, a renewed faith began to develop. She also grew in compassion and understanding for others. We talked about the medications she'd taken over the last several months and their negative side effects, particularly those that altered her ability to read and process information. That a chemical change could so profoundly affect intellect baffled her, and she realized that she was experiencing what people with learning disabilities endure their entire lives. Her perspective changed.

As a little girl, Chloe often asked why other students were slow to learn things, why they didn't understand concepts that, to her, were basic. We spent many afternoons talking about the differences in each of us, and the fact that she possessed a mind that worked quickly. It often felt like I was talking to a wall. She honestly believed that people with learning difficulties didn't try hard. Now she got it. Through her own experience, she realized that much of what we take for granted, or assume credit for, is a genetic luck-of-the-draw.

From my journal: "Chloe's eighteenth birthday. I can't believe it. Such a milestone. We're so proud of her. I am especially impressed with how well she's doing despite the challenges. She is an inspiration. I love her dearly.

"Eighteen years ago Mark and I were at the hospital, laboring away. We didn't know that in sixteen hours, a perfect little girl would come into our world. She is perfect. I can't imagine life without her, without the depth and character she adds to my existence, to the experience of my soul. She's a blessing—one of many. My gratitude runs deep."

I still feel this way, probably even more than when I wrote those words. Surprisingly, the vastness of my gratitude for Chloe, her illness, and all that it encompasses would fill an ocean. Our shared experiences transformed us. I'm a much better person for having traveled this journey. I accept situations as they are, and seek from them knowledge and growth. I've learned to initiate change lovingly, rather than forcefully, and to realize that my timetable might not be another's. I've learned how deceiving appearances can be. Thanks to strange, unbelievable moments I've experienced, I try not to judge others. I've moved closer to the soul I want to be. Incongruently, I wouldn't have progressed point had the route been smoother. I'd smugly have thought that I knew the way without seeking direction.

My feelings were not always this rosy. Shortly after Chloe's birthday, her mood and demeanor deteriorated again. Having experienced a stretch of "nearly normal" days, I was surprised when she plunged into rapid cycles of irritability, anger, melancholy, sleeplessness, depression, and grandiosity. When Chloe didn't sleep, I stayed up too, not knowing what she might do while manic. Since Mark had to go to work early in the morning, I tried not to change his routine, or awaken him. I still felt like this was my job.

As silly as it sounds, I also wanted to protect Mark from Chloe's illness. His mom's mental illness drastically altered his childhood and teen years, and I sought to spare him these similar experiences. My controlling personality was seriously at work here, and in many ways, I again became a martyr, determined to shoulder it all and "bear up" under the pressure.

I subconsciously set myself up as the sole responsible party for Chloe's well-being. I had some sort of savior complex, because I wrongly thought that if I made all the right decisions and did all the right things, she would be healthy and well. I assumed, as a parent, if I did everything right, everything would be all right. The problem was, how could I figure out what was right?

Many people must feel this way as they begin parenting. We think we're all powerful, all knowing. We think we have control over the outcomes of our children's lives. I've learned better, but it took a long time and many "learning opportunities" to do so. My perspective now is this: As parents, we set examples and teach core values that our children will rely on for their entire lives. Most significantly, we teach them about unconditional love, respect for self and others, hope, faith, acceptance and tolerance. However, that does not mean their lives will be perfect, or easy, or even, by commonly held assumptions, good. They, we, have lessons to learn. Soul refinements are achievements, often through great challenge.

We must love and support one another through it all. That is not to say we must accept behaviors that don't mesh with our values, but if we are to achieve our highest level of being, we must love freely, despite those behaviors. Nevertheless, these realizations were hard-won.

Before I truly accepted our situation, I worked hard to manage it. Academically, through research and study, and physically, by applying what I was learning, I tried to stay on top of it. I was determined to be in control, or at least knowledgeable. I held unrealistic expectations for myself, and they bled into other areas of my life. I expected too much of Michael and Monica, wanting them to adapt their behavior to Chloe's needs. Of course, this was ridiculous, since her responses were neither predictable nor normal, and they often wondered what I wanted them to do, how I wanted them to be.

As the burden became too heavy and fatigue again took its toll, I began again to grieve and beg for the grace to get through each day. We soon understood why most families of the mentally ill fall apart, why divorce is common when children suffer long-term or life-threatening illness.

The pressures of chronic illness, laid atop the challenges of raising a family, exhaust everybody. When we're tired all the time, unless we remain aware of our attitudes and behaviors, we mistreat those closest to us. Lost sleep, challenging medical and parenting decisions, and pure grief resulting from releasing my ideals of perfection led me down the lane of blame.

For the first time in our married life, I resented Mark, despite the fact that he was doing his best to support, empathize, and buoy me up. I resented him working outside our home, while I handled the situation within. I envied his legitimate escape from the difficult details of raising children and dealing with chronic illness, as I developed tunnel vision and thought of "the cure," and little else. It took years for me to accept the illness rather than try to cure or change it. Without acceptance, I continued to be engulfed by waves of unrealistic hope that ultimately came crashing down.

I rarely held a conversation that didn't focus on Bipolar Disorder or a related topic. My persistence on the subject drove Mark nuts and only occasionally did he stop my carrying-on. One evening, as I narrated a blow-by-blow of the day's symptoms and incidents, and my reactions, he stopped me.

"I know you need to talk about this, Katie, but I don't want to hear it. I do not need every single detail. Just do what you have to do, and tell me what you want me to do to help her get better."

This was not what I wanted to hear. I wanted Mark to know the details of my difficult days, wanted him to share my grief. I wanted him to understand how hard my situation was, commiserate with me, and offer up some helpful suggestions. If he couldn't do that, I at least wanted him to sympathize and encourage me, tell me I was doing a good job. I wanted recognition for my hard work, acknowledgement of my sacrifices. I didn't get what I wanted. I wasn't happy about that.

Again, my journal verifies that these were not my proudest days. My ability to cope fluctuated, at times completely eluded me. 29 March 2000: "I grieve. There is so much loss, from simple and short term to complex and far-reaching. I cry over the loss of my daily life, my routine. I miss time to myself, a pace of my own, and freedom to spend my days as I like. I yearn for quiet, serenity, and peace. I have ten to twelve hours a week in which to accomplish what I must and replenish my dwindling inner resources.

"When Chloe is home noise, tension, and contrariness rule. She plays music so loudly the neighbors can hear it through closed doors and windows. She refuses to let anyone else watch a TV show or choose an activity. Because she's sick, she thinks her needs and wants are more important than everything else's. It doesn't matter if someone is trying to sleep, or study, or talk on the phone, she's compelled to create distractions to escape her inner noise. Despite knowing this, my jaw is firm, my teeth clenched. My temples ache from unreleased tension. I am frightened. I am angry. I do not like *me* right now.

"As soon as Monica and Michael get home from school the discord begins. Chloe cannot be nice to them, and perpetual bickering or giddy, noisy, aggressiveness permeate our home. It takes more inner resources than I have left to get through each afternoon. I'm emotionally and physically exhausted. How will I keep this up?

"I miss so many things I always took for granted. I miss time alone with Mark. I miss looking forward to the time when we can travel together. I miss my life and the plans I had made for it. Mark must think I'm selfish. Or do *I* think I'm selfish? I know this is a huge burden for Chloe, but it's a challenge for all of us — for me. Mark leaves every day, and enjoys his own life, separate from this. He calls Chloe every day, and no longer checks in with me. (I sound like a jealous schoolgirl.) She adores her dad and saves her negativity for me. I'm doing the hard stuff, and getting the lousy treatment.

"Mark's never filled a prescription, never made an appointment, never documented symptoms, and never explained any of this to Michael and Monica. He has never gone to the mental hospital, or taken her to an office visit. He's never listened to her 'detached from reality' conversations, never heard Michael and Monica voice fears, and concerns. He's never called the school, never attended a teacher conference, and never done homework with her. He's never taken a razor or a straight pin from her firm grasp, never seen her bloody arms. He's never heard her weep and beg for death. He has reserved for himself the role of provider and abdicated to me the responsibility of caretaker. Okay. Wait. I'm the one who engineered these roles. But I sure don't like it now."

Obviously, the role I'd assumed didn't turn out to be the one for which I'd prepared. I was in over my head, barely staying afloat. I sometimes fantasized about a life where I remained in the workforce and Mark and I met these medical challenges together. Even in those fantasies, I was the responsible party. I made this choice, and now it required me to learn new skills, new practices, and new "ways to be." However, that intellectual understanding didn't always convince my aching heart and racing mind.

"GOD. I know he agonizes, but we need to redefine our roles or life as we know it, as a couple, will be over. I fear that possibility, knowing it's conceivable. We're losing sight of one another as partners, a consequence I cannot accept. We need to be a team. I must find balance between my needs and my family's...and so must Mark.

"Oh. There is so much with this thing."

Mark and I had so much to learn. Further complicating those lessons, Chloe entered the hospital four days later.

18

April 2000

"Sometimes to live is an act of courage."
— Lucius Annaeus Seneca

As my journal indicated, Chloe unraveled. Visions of walking through sliding glass doors and throwing herself through windows tormented her. Plagued by whispers and muffled voices, she dared not be alone and refused any quiet place where the noises in her head came into focus. The physical tension and emotional anxiety grew so intense she took warm mineral-salt baths every two or three hours in an attempt to alleviate them. When this failed, she began cutting her arms again to feel temporary relief, or release, or maybe just as a distraction. In fearful anticipation of the violent and bloody scenes that assaulted her dreams, she avoided sleep. Her hands shook, her speech was rapid and pressured, and she was perpetually tearful. This went on for days.

Exhausted and paranoid, Chloe thought everything her brother and sister said or did was negative and directed at her. She assaulted them with words and attitude. By Saturday night she couldn't sleep, consumed by the deep distress and anxiety of simultaneous depression and mania, often called a "mixed state."

Earlier in the day Dr. Kahil recommended medication changes, but warned me, she might not be "safe" and that I should consider a brief hospitalization. I didn't want to do that, yet could not risk leaving her alone. She had to be within sight. I even followed her to the bathroom, hovering outside the door, listening for anything suspicious. I stayed with her all night, knowing she'd reached her limit and saw suicide as a blessed release.

During those dark hours, we talked little and cried a lot. Since hugging or touching sometimes irritated Chloe, we were fortunate that physical contact comforted her at this time. She lay on the sofa with her head in my lap as I stroked her hair and rubbed her arms and back. Then she would shift to sit next to me, with her head on my shoulder, and I would wrap my arms around her and gently rock. In many ways, it was time blissfully spent. I consoled her. The process soothed my heart.

The warm comfort of unconditional love enveloped us as a relative calm descended and provided a sense of safety for a little while. As parent and child, we lovingly got through the night, knowing we were en route to uncharted territory. On Sunday, we agreed she needed to be in the hospital. She couldn't promise that she wouldn't hurt herself and I couldn't continue this round-the-clock vigil.

It was difficult to tell Mark that Chloe needed to be in the hospital. He, we, had seen his mom in a mental hospital many times and it was always a painful experience. When she passed away, as much as he grieved her absence, he was happy that she no longer suffered the symptoms of her illness. She was finally at peace, free. My heart ached for him as we talked about it and his eyes welled up, but refused to flow over.

Mark is a fix-it man, a problem solver. He's accustomed to making things "right," but this was a rare instance when "right" could not be made. I wished he didn't have to go through this again.

When she was ready, Mark and I drove Chloe to the hospital and filled out the paperwork. Because she was eighteen, she signed herself in. We requested that she stay in the pediatric ward, and since Dr. Kahil agreed, the hospital staff complied

We accompanied Chloe through a series of secured doors, to the reception desk of the pediatric psychiatric ward. At the desk, we handed over the few things she brought with her. The nursing staff looked through the bag and removed her childhood blanket and portable CD player with earphones.

We had to take them home since they were potential suicide devices. She could have the rest of her things in twenty-four to forty-eight hours. Then they asked us to say goodbye and leave with a nurse who escorted us out. I hugged Chloe tightly, told her I loved her, and I would see her tomorrow. She looked back at me with the deepest sadness a child's eyes can convey, tears silently sliding down her cheeks.

Once out of Chloe's sight, grief and fear consumed me. Uncontrollable sobs wracked by body. I couldn't take another step for fear of falling; my legs trembled and felt like jelly. Tightness gripped my chest and waves of nausea washed over me. My palpable sorrow ran deeper than I could have imagined. I was physically ill, ached all over. Mark held me in that hallway as I struggled to regain my composure. A tear slid down the nurse's cheek as she cooed, "I know, honey. I know. It's so hard to be a mama."

I did not want Chloe in the hospital, but that was where she needed to be. I did not want to leave, but was not allowed to stay. I did not want her to be sick, but she was. I did not want her to suffer from a chronic mental illness, but she most certainly did.

19

April/May 2000

"Tolerance and celebration of individual differences is the fire that fuels lasting love."
— Tom Hannah

"I brought Chloe home today."

After only four days in the hospital, Chloe came home. Thanks to her brief stay were able to rest and refocus our energies on getting well rather than surviving the night. It also gave Mark and me a few days to talk to Monica and Michael about Chloe's illness and its behavioral and social ramifications. These were tough to understand.

A destabilized mood disorder changes one's personality and the manner in which that person interacts with others. This factor alone makes it hard to live and get along with someone diagnosed with Bipolar Disorder. It's even harder when you're a sibling living and dealing with the unpredictability and irrationality day after day.

People with Bipolar Disorder often experience paranoia and anxiety, which manifest as irritability. Chloe regularly lost patience and yelled at the others for being too noisy when they laughed or played, exuding sounds of joy. When they talked to her, she responded sharply, so they stopped talking. Her depression translated into grumpy intolerance, which Michael and Monica were tired of enduring.

In my reading, I learned that destabilized patients with Bipolar Disorder are frequently egocentric, and Chloe definitely was. Michael and Monica grew intolerant of her demands and expectations. They were tired of giving up the computer when she wanted it, tired of watching shows she chose, and tired of eating food she preferred. They were tired of name-calling if they didn't understand something she tried to explain, and of criticism of everything from what they wore to their choice of friends. She took out her frustrations on our immediate family, and the other children were fed up. We all lost patience. We needed to develop greater tolerance. It was time for Monica and Michael to know more about the illness, and I wanted to share as much information as possible without dramatizing or inciting fear. Mostly, I wanted them to love, accept, and support their sister unconditionally. Sometimes it seemed like I wanted the world.

When someone you love is chronically ill, separating the person from the illness is challenging. Relinquishing judgment and unreasonable expectations of accountability seem impossible. Unless the one with illness is stable, we must cultivate understanding. It wasn't that I didn't expect Chloe to be accountable for the things she said and did, but her perception of reality was sometimes different from the perceptions of those around her. Unless she was healthy, the rest of us needed to know that she might do and say things that seemed inappropriate.

We had to make an effort not to take things personally. Over time, I expected her to learn to manage her illness, and to treat others respectfully despite how she felt. However, developing these skills would require time with a therapist, and a high degree of introspection. When one is fighting to stay alive, introspection and personal growth seem rather esoteric. The rest of us needed to learn new skills first. Therefore, we tried to do that, and Chloe came home to siblings who knew more about the details of her illness and were willing to work at getting along.

On increased doses of five different medications, Chloe was finally able to sleep. However, sleeping well quickly transmuted into oversleeping, and she could not wake up for school. Between hospitalization and transition time at home, she missed two full weeks.

Fortunately, her mind cleared in the afternoon, allowing her to study and work on the assignments that her teachers sent home without question. Neither of us ever anticipated this finale to her grandly successful high school years, but we were taking life one day at a time without focusing on what might have been.

At our next meeting with Dr. Kahil, I asked about the amount of sleep Chloe now seemed to require. He explained.

"Chloe's brain is recovering from prolonged chemical and electrical trauma. It is as real as a physical injury and she needs sleep to heal. It could be months before she sleeps less. Don't wake her up for school. She'll catch up. For now, sleep and recovery are more important than anything else."

Again, I was surprised. How long would it take me to understand? Unrealistically, I considered graduation and the accompanying activities ultimately important, without considering how sick Chloe was. My ability to deny amazed even me.

For the duration of her senior year, Chloe maintained a semblance of stability. She slept a lot, occasionally made it to class, and completed all the assigned work in her two classes. In May of 2000, she proudly took her place among the top scholars in her graduating class. Glowing, she mingled with fellow graduates and enjoyed friends who came to support her, knowing she'd achieved something monumental under difficult circumstances. I never felt greater pride than I felt for her that night.

After the ceremony, a large crowd congregated on the field. Conversations overlapped as graduates called out to friends on the opposite side of the field and parents talked to folks they hadn't seen in months. Noisy chatter surrounded us and Chloe handled it well. No anxiety. No feelings of panic. No temptation to cry. No problem. Her optimism and ebullience swelled. She got through the evening with emotions and reactions not unlike the other graduates. Feeling centered and confident, she mingled with classmates, taking photographs and sharing moments accentuated by hugs and kisses, laughter and joy.

I encouraged her when she asked about hanging out with fellow graduates. She deserved to have fun in the company of friends she had not seen for so long. My heart swelled with love and gratitude for the normalcy as Chloe headed out in her own car while Mark, Michael, Monica, and I went home.

Once there, we settled in for a quiet night. Basking in the aura of the evening, Mark and I snuggled on the sofa, chatting, watching television, and reflecting on the milestone we'd just passed. Michael and Monica were busy with their own activities, and made no demands on our time or attention. Although pleasantly normal, the evening felt unique and supreme. Had we not experienced the past few months' events, this precious evening would have seemed ordinary.

The human organism, like the entire natural world, takes the path of least resistance. Without hardship, our true selves, our interiors, our souls if you will, fail to grow. Of course, we all know people who seem to have horrible luck and never get a break. Repeatedly, these people struggle and suffer. We look on and wonder why. As onlookers, we have no notion of the internal transformations taking place. Trials provide the opportunity to choose. We can choose learning, growth, acceptance, and peace. Or we can choose stubborn resistance, cling to our current state, and repeatedly experience similar trials. Mark and I chose to grow together, and were learning to appreciate the beauty of the mundane, the value of what we used to take for granted. We recognized and reveled in the joy, no matter how short-lived.

We heard Chloe come in long before eleven o'clock and assumed she wanted to change clothes or pick up something she'd forgotten. One look at her face told us something was terribly wrong. Mascara-stained trails of tears ran down her cheeks, puddling on her neck and chest. Her sorrowful eyes, swollen and red, silently told of the sobs that had earlier wracked her body. My heart sank to join hers as I wrapped my arms around her shoulders and sought an explanation.

After talking to several classmates, Chloe heard where her friends were gathering and thought she'd meet up with her old crowd and go over together. Her arrival at Jade's house was a surprise, since Laura, Sammy, and Jade had not hung out with Chloe since Winter Formal.

The weeks turned into months, and the foursome comfortably evolved into a threesome. The girls smiled, hugged, and greeted Chloe. Like old times, the four of them chatted while getting ready to go out. In what seemed like the normal course of things, Chloe found herself alone in Jade's room. Moments later, when the other three returned together, she knew something was askew.

Sammy walked in ahead of the others and, without hesitation, said, "Chloe, not to be mean or anything, but we don't want you to go out with us."

Hurt and surprised, Chloe asked, "What do you mean you don't want me to go? Why not? It'll be fun."

Jade looked away, detaching herself from the situation, while Laura stepped up behind Sammy, providing encouragement and support to the spokeswoman.

"We don't want to hang out with you. It's not like we're still friends or anything. You've hardly been around and we're, like, not comfortable having you with us. Besides, I don't think they want you at the parties we're going to."

Chloe looked at Jade, who was once her best friend, for help. There was none. Then she got angry. "You know I've been sick. How can you do this to me? How can you be so mean? Jade, you know what it's been like for me. You know what I've been through, but I'm getting better. It'll be fun. It will." She begged, "Why aren't you on my side?"

Nothing.

As Chloe continued to plead, Sammy strengthened her resolve to go without her.

"We're embarrassed to be with you, Chloe. You're not one of us any more. You should hear what people are saying. They think you're crazy or a druggie. Some kids are afraid to have you around 'cuz they don't know what you might do or say. I even heard that some parents think you're pregnant because you're, well…bigger."

The rumors had run rampant, and from the retelling, it seemed to me, Laura and Sammy got a certain high out of revealing them to Chloe. They dredged up the times she'd made irrational or unreasonable comments, trying to justify their unkindness. Jade stood mute through it all.

"Chloe," Laura said, "nobody wants you there. It's bad. If we show up with you, they might not let us in. We're not gonna let you ruin our graduation night."

Because Chloe had been close to the family hosting the first party they were planning to hit and assumed they had a fondness for her, this was the final blow. She believed what turned out to be lies and distortions, and felt like she didn't have an ally in the world. The verbal barrage hit its target, destroying her confidence.

In the end, a hysterical Chloe verbally assaulted the trio. "You fucking bitches. I can't believe we were ever friends. You're such assholes. You have no clue. No clue."

She ran to her car, jumped in, and raced up the highway toward the mountains, planning to drive over the side. Then she had a change of heart, turned around, and careened down the dark road toward home and safety.

So there we were, drowning in sorrow at the end of a day that had shown so much promise, held such joy. This day was a microcosm of Chloe's life, a roller coaster of rapidly changing emotions over which she had little control. The trauma was profound and she retreated into a childlike state. I helped her out of her clothes and into her pajamas, and then washed her face and neck with a cool cloth.

As Chloe began to settle down, the phone rang. It was David, one of her best friends. She was still upset enough to cry as she explained what happened while he listened supportively. Then he told her to get out of bed and get her party clothes back on, he and "the other" David were coming over. Within thirty minutes, the Davids arrived to take Chloe out for a night of graduation fun. I love them for being such good friends. They cared for her then, as they do now, deeply and profoundly. What wonderful, compassionate people.

My anger toward Jade, Laura, and Sammy, though fleeting, was dangerously powerful. It seethed and threatened to boil over, held at bay only by my commitment to letting go of judgment and accepting what was. I probably also felt comfort in having someone else to blame for Chloe's ills.

Months later, when I ran into the girls at the coffee shop, and again at the mall, I never mentioned that night. It took discipline not to confront them, not to make them aware of the pain they'd inflicted. Nevertheless, my heart reminded me that they were just girls, uninformed and frightened, and terribly young. Faced with the powerful truth that one of their own was stricken, they retreated in blind fear. I understand that reaction, but I also know that when people in the world are right and balanced, compassion flows in both directions. I want to add to, not take from, that rightness and balance.

20
Summer 2000

"The harder the conflict, the more glorious the triumph. What we obtain too cheap, we esteem too lightly. It is dearness only that gives everything its value. I love the man that can smile in trouble that can gather strength from distress and grow brave by reflection. 'Tis the business of little minds to shrink; but he whose heart is firm, and whose conscience approves his conduct, will pursue his principles unto death."

— Thomas Paine

It took a couple of weeks for Chloe to recover from the humiliation and disappointment she felt on graduation night. She slept a lot and saw only a few friends—all boys—who accepted her as she was. She continued going to Maria, to whom she had returned for therapy, and talked to her on the phone between visits. She became more actively involved during her appointments with Dr. Kahil and made an effort to manage her medications without my reminders. She began to feel better and the emotional shroud that had enveloped her for so long loosened just a bit.

We enjoyed a lull that lasted for several weeks. We took a couple of family vacations, Chloe spent a week in California with my mom, and Monica and Michael took trips with friends. Chloe felt so much better, in fact, that she began a part time job and made plans to move into an honor's dorm at the University in August. The only downturn in her illness occurred mid-July, when she stopped sleeping, became irritable, and began spending more money than she had. Dr. Kahil recognized the classic symptoms of emerging mania and doubled her mood stabilizer. Within a couple of weeks, she was back in control.

I encouraged Chloe to prepare for college and hoped for her success, but I prepared myself for the possibility that this

Kate L. McLaughlin

venture into the world was much too soon. I vacillated between feeling confident that she was stable and that she would never get bad again, and thinking that a hospitalization was just around the corner if she was not careful. I wanted to keep things in perspective and appreciate steps forward, while preparing for the likelihood of relapse. I had not yet learned I was not in control, life is full of surprises, and those surprises make living the ultimate adventure.

Mark shared my uncertainty about Chloe's wellness and ability to move into the dorm and start at the university. Several things led us to wonder about, and sometimes doubt, the wisdom of her moving out. The biggest concern was that she still did not manage her own medication. It was the rare day when she took all of her meds without a reminder. She still took them because we wanted her to, and not because she needed them to be well. What would happen if I were not there to prod her?

We also worried because I was the instigator for the paperwork and registration activities prerequisite to enrollment. She did everything I asked her to do, but initiated nothing. She would have done these things without my involvement if she were truly ready for university. Should I back off? Should we discourage going to college for now? Alternatively, should we continue to move forward as if she had never been ill in order to give her the best platform from which to jump? Finally, instead of questioning and assuming, I approached Chloe about my concerns. We spoke frankly.

"Mom, I don't want to have Bipolar Disorder. I don't want to take my medicine, but I know I have to, so I will. I'm mad that I can't go to NYU or USC because of this thing, but I want to go to school. My brain is working right again. I can handle the school stuff. The social stuff scares me, but that scares everybody who first goes to college. I want to be a normal college freshman. I want to move on and put this crap behind me. It doesn't define me. I won't let it. I don't want my roommate to know. I don't want anybody to know."

"You'll have to share some of it with your roommate, Chloe. You'll be in a very small space together. Eventually she'll see your meds and figure out that something's going on. And what if you get bad? It'll be scary if she doesn't know anything and doesn't know what to do. You don't have to tell her right away, but she'll need to know sooner rather than later."

"I know. I'll tell her as much as I have to, and I'll make sure she has your phone number in case something happens. But I don't think it will. I think the worst is over. I'm going to be okay."

Our candid conversation soothed us both, and as July turned to August, she jumped into college preparations. She took her meds without reminders, and made her own refill requests at the pharmacy. She wrote lists of things she needed for school, and the two of us shopped for dorm and school supplies. She was content and excited.

My journal reads: "We passed through a challenging period, emerging better for the experience. I count my blessings daily. Yes—there have been hardships, but they have made life interesting and fine. They've spawned growth, creativity, and gratitude. We will always have problems of one sort or another (everybody does), but we have the abilities and skills to solve them, grow personally, and develop spiritually and emotionally. Myriad possibilities exist when we're open to opportunity and potential, as well as grace, and love, and inspiration. Without times of challenge, we fail to recognize the bounty."

Feeling strongly about this truth, I proceeded, as usual, into scholarly mode and searched for others who might eloquently have voiced the same understanding. I found myself in excellent company. Perhaps my favorite affirmation came in the form of a fortune cookie whose telling slip of paper I taped to my computer desk. It reads, "He who does not taste the bitter cannot enjoy the sweet."

We had, indeed, tasted the bitter, and now yearned to enjoy the sweet. As all of us hoped for the best, on Thursday, August 17th, in the year 2000, eighteen-year-old Chloe moved into an honors dorm at the university to begin her undergraduate experience.

She was excited about being on her own, having control over her time and calendar, and meeting new people. She enjoyed making her small room feel cozy and spent hours selecting bed linens and décor. When we got to the dorm, her roommate was there and ready to settle in.

We carted an incredible amount of stuff up the steps and down the hall, and the girls found ingenious ways to make it all fit. Since they'd talked on the phone several times, coordinating what each of them would bring, their room came together nicely and looked like a comfortable little home.

For the next several days, Chloe prepared for the first day of school. She bought books and supplies, located classrooms, learned how to use her student I.D./debit card, and attended orientation meetings. She called several times a day, always happy and excited, eager to share new information, and perpetually upbeat. Each time I got off the phone, I felt encouraged. I thought that maybe we had this thing licked. Maybe the worst was behind her and the future would be sweet.

21
Fall 2000

"Learn to adjust yourself to the conditions you have to endure, but make a point of trying to alter or correct conditions so that they are most favorable to you."
  —William Frederick Book

I must have been greatly relieved with Chloe settled at the dorm, because for months I wrote nothing but revisions on my first book. I had faithfully kept a journal for most of my life, so I surprise myself when I look back through my notebooks and find not a word from mid-September through December. I recall feeling the same glorious freedom I'd felt when Monica started school and I had a few hours each day to myself.

This sense of independence felt even more precious since I'd had it, lost it, and got it back again. I felt happily relieved of the burden of caring for a mentally-ill child. I was thrilled to forget, if only for a time, that such was even the case. I know that I talked to her every day, sometimes more than once a day. I also remember driving to the university at least once a week to see her. Sometimes she was well, sometimes not. A daily log of the details simply does not exist. However, other documentation does.

My reading list for that year is evidence that Bipolar Disorder persisted as an underlying focus. I have long kept track of the books I read, giving each one a rating from one to five. The titles listed for the fall of 2000 included: Sylvia Plath's *The Bell Jar, Mrs. Dalloway* by Virginia Wolf, *A Brilliant Madness* by Patty Duke, and *An Unquiet Mind, Touched With Fire,* and *Night Falls Fast* by Kay Redfield Jamison, as well as several medical texts on the subject. Of course, I also read books for pleasure, but was definitely preoccupied with finding the cause, finding a "cure," learning to live with mental illness.

Although I lacked my usual written account of events, the calendar and a large envelope of materials I had collected and saved from that time told the tale. I returned to my regular volunteer position at the University Extension Office and our family participated in weekly volleyball games. I continued to get Monica and Michael to soccer practices, games, and tournaments. Work and social obligations returned to the schedule, and I even had time to meet with my editor, publisher, and illustrator a few times.

From mid-August through October, I took Chloe for blood work every other week and to Dr. Kahil about every ten days. She saw Maria nearly as often. Almost weekly notes reminded me to pick up new prescriptions, indicating that she was not stable and that Dr. Kahil was continually changing her meds. The calendar also attested to a life much like it was before mental illness intruded.

In many ways, we reverted to old routines when Chloe moved into the dorm. Mark and I resumed regular date nights. Michael and Monica invited friends over again. A feeling of heaviness lifted, and all of us felt relieved to have the source of so much turmoil removed from our immediate environment. Then other shadowy issues snuck into our family picture.

Stronger and more energetic following the mono, Michael began to feel the void of sports in his life. While his friends continued to work out and train through the summer and fall of 2000, he developed new friends with different interests. He drank on the weekends and smoked pot after school. His grades were still good, but his attitude and demeanor changed over a period of months. He slept later and later on the weekends, and I heard a rumor that he was drunk at the high school football games.

Of course, I couldn't verify those rumors and in all honesty, I didn't try to. I was in denial about Michael's potential for disaster. My attention was focused on keeping Chloe healthy.

As a Fine Arts/Studio Art major, Chloe took two art classes her first semester. Her work amazed me. I knew she was artistic, had known since she won a countywide art contest at age five, but I never really appreciated the depth of her talent. When she shared sketches she'd made in her figure drawing class, it was like looking at the model through a black and white lens. The details and nuances enthralled me. She produced realistic drawings with little effort and no thought, making it seem like the easiest thing in the world. She looked and she drew, producing incredible results. The fact that many artists also suffered from Bipolar Disorder was not lost on either of us. In fact, we sometimes wondered if stability meant a change in creativity. Of course, stability remained an elusive goal.

Chloe's roommate Caitlyn, a kind and patient young woman who remains her friend to this day, called me a few weeks into the semester.

"Mrs. McLaughlin, I didn't know if I should call you or not, but I'm worried about Chloe."

"Caitlyn, if you're worried, then I'm glad you called. What's going on?"

"Well, Chloe hardly ever gets out of bed. When I leave for class in the morning, she's there, and when I come home in the afternoon, it looks like she hasn't moved. She's not going to class, and she's not eating. I don't know what to do."

"You were right to call. I'll talk to her, maybe take her back to the doctor. Thanks, Caitlyn."

"It's okay. I just hope Chloe won't be mad that I called you."

"I don't think she will. She'll know you're worried about her. Please call me any time you have concerns or questions."

I got off the phone and tried to reach Chloe on her cell. When she didn't answer, I left a message, then called Dr. Kahil for an appointment and waited for her to call me back.

That evening when I talked to Chloe, she assured me that, although Caitlyn's reports were true, she was staying on top of her coursework and was not falling behind. When I met her in front of her dorm the next day, I was grateful that Caitlyn had called me. Chloe looked sullen and sad. Her head hung down and her eyes drooped along with the corners of her mouth. Her hair was stringy and she wore no makeup. She clearly needed a medication adjustment.

A couple weeks later Caitlyn called again to say that Chloe's depression seemed to be deepening, and wondered if there was anything she should do. She asked about Bipolar

Disorder, and peppered me with a list of well-thought-out questions. Chloe, by this time, had offered a general explanation of her illness, and what it meant, but Caitlyn wanted to know more. I answered her questions and suggested some resources, encouraging her to call anytime.

"You know, Mrs. McLaughlin, I really like Chloe. We get along and we're good roommates, but I never thought I'd be living with someone with such serious problems. Sometimes it bothers me. I had all these ideas about what my roommate and I would do together, and what dorm life and college would be like. It's not what I thought it would be. But I want to help. I want to learn what I can, do what I can. I hope you don't mind if I call and ask questions."

As Caitlyn spoke frankly about her feelings, fears, and disappointments, I became acquainted with her good heart and accepting nature. I knew then that Chloe had been very lucky. Caitlyn was the best roommate she could have had. Her maturity, strong sense of self, and lack of judgment made that difficult semester bearable. I count Caitlyn as one of many blessings we received as a direct result of Chloe's illness.

My November 2000 calendar documents significant change. Chloe saw Dr. Kahil every week and I crossed off many commitments from the weekly pages because she was not well and needed me. November 15th was such a day. CHLOE ILL was scrawled across the calendar page in bold red letters, reminding me of the dramatic events.

I was at the Extension Office when Chloe called me, not sounding at all right. Initially, her voice indicated flat affect and detachment. She told me she did not feel good and wanted me to come get her and take her home. I tried to talk her into staying on campus and going to class, or at least staying until I finished my shift. She became hysterical. She cried and shouted into the phone.

"I'm not going to class today. I might not ever go again. How do you expect me to worry about going to a stupid class when all I can think about is dying and how to accomplish that? I need you to come get me. I need you to come get me NOW."

"Chloe, listen to me."

Sobbing, she interrupted, "Just forget it, Mom. Don't come. I'm fine. I am fine. I'll take care of myself. I don't want you here. I do not want to be here. I'm sorry. I'm sorry. I won't ever do this again. I can't keep doing this. I can't do this any more."

"Chloe, I'll be there as soon as I can, but you have to promise me you won't do anything to hurt yourself before I get there."

"I can't. I can't make that promise."

Afraid to hang up the phone, needing to remain connected, I pleaded, "Chloe, I know this is hard. I know you don't want to feel this way, but please try to have faith that you'll feel better soon. You've felt this bad before and you got better. You'll get better again. We just need to get you to the doctor and change your medication."

"I'm sick of medication. I'm sick of changing it. He can't fix me, Mom. Don't you get it? I cannot be fixed. I will always be this way. I don't want to do it any more."

We went round and round for what seemed like a very long time. It took some effort to settle Chloe to a point where I thought she would be safe if we hung up. I told her how much we all loved her and would do whatever it took to help her get well. I assured her it would be okay, that she would feel better soon. I soothed her with words, wishing she could feel my touch through the telephone line.

During this conversation, a fellow volunteer sat at the next desk, listening to the entire exchange. I'd told very few people about Chloe's health and to those, I'd shared no details. Being overheard made me uncomfortable, but Chloe's sheer distress overshadowed those concerns as I calmly coaxed her to hold on, I'd be there in fifteen minutes. I got off the phone, made my apologies, and headed down to the university, silently praying that she wouldn't do anything to hurt herself before I got there.

I brought Chloe home, where she stayed much of the remainder of the fall term. I cleared my calendar and again focused on getting all three children where they needed to be, when they needed to be there. My publisher and I agreed that we would pick up the book promotion after the first of the year and I officially resigned from my volunteer duties. I fit holiday preparations into available hours, and saw friends when time permitted. We adapted to the demands of our situation, and finally, I was able to remain calm and relatively unruffled when plans had to change. One of the most valuable lessons I learned during this time was to be truly flexible by reprioritizing and adjusting to ever-evolving needs.

A few times after I brought her home, Chloe spent the night in her dorm room, but anxiety inevitably forced her back home. Like months before, she no longer wanted to socialize or participate in extra-curricular activities. She spent most of her time in her pajamas, and hours in the bathtub, trying desperately to ease the tension, anxiety, and discomfort. She was not well enough to drive, so I took her to and from school and appointments. She saw Dr. Kahil and Maria weekly. She was getting worse instead of better.

Despite the severity of her illness and Dr. Kahil's unsuccessful attempts to stabilize her, Chloe got through finals. Like other students in the dorms, she moved her personal things home for winter break, leaving her computer and other large items stacked on the bed so the floors could be cleaned. All along, I assumed she would recuperate through the holidays and return to the dorm and college routine when the spring semester opened in mid-January.

22
Holidays 2000

"... in health the genial pretence must be kept up, and the effort
renewed — to communicate, to civilize, to share, to cultivate the desert,
to educate the native, to work together by day and by night to sport. In
illness this make-believe ceases."
— Virginia Woolf

The holidays were blessedly uneventful. We did very
little outside our immediate family, but still enjoyed the
season. Chloe began babysitting again for a family whose
children she adored. She spent many hours there, and was
able to hold things together quite well. Aside from that,
however, she had few interests or activities. She continued
seeing both Maria and Dr. Kahil weekly. Mark and I hoped
for the best.

Winter break passed quickly. Though still enrolled in
several courses and committed to her dorm room, Chloe did
not want to go back to school. We talked about it and decided
she could ease into classes the first week, then move back to
campus when she adjusted to her schedule. On the first day of
class she panicked, she couldn't go. Within days, she didn't
sleep. The unraveling happened so quickly that we were in
crisis before I realized it and called Dr. Kahil.

He added another medication, calling in the prescription
to the pharmacy, and explaining to me over the phone how
gradually to increase the dose to avoid negative reactions. I
jotted his instructions on my calendar, which bears witness to
the ensuing panic in other ways, too. Every few days "Call Dr.
Kahil" is scribbled into slots provided for appointments, and
many scheduled activities are lined out, missed despite having
been calendared. Many "to do" lists include calling to cancel
one commitment or another.

One week's calendar margins contain details that I must
have related to the doctor over the phone. They were written in
two hands: Chloe's and mine.

> "Requires more sleep
> Falls to sleep more easily
> Can't wake up
> Doesn't want to be alone
> Voice quivers
> Hands shake
> Anxious about weight gain
> More anxiety in general
> Forgetful
> Distractible
> Rapidly shifting moods"

An appointment with the bursar's office finalized her
medically necessitated withdrawal from school during this same
week. It was not an easy time.

The following week I made an appointment for myself with
Dr. Kahil. I always went with her to the doctor, so nothing was
secret from me, but I wanted to talk to him on my own. I wanted
the opportunity to explore my questions and fears without
concern over how Chloe would react. I wanted to know the
practical details of what we were dealing with. In truth, I was
scared and frustrated and needed some assurance or
encouragement.

He scheduled me at the end of office hours and spent a long
time explaining Chloe's treatment and prognosis. Having
thoroughly researched the topic, I was already familiar with
general explanations and information. That is not what I wanted.
I wanted to know his opinion of the severity of her illness. Had
he treated others like her? What was their progress like? Did he
think she would be able to return to school? Why had the
medications not worked thus far? What would he try next?
Would she ever function independently? How were we going to
keep her alive?

How were we going to keep her alive?

I left Dr. Kahil's office with a lot to consider. He frankly
admitted that she was one of the most difficult cases he had

treated, but not the worst. She was an ultra-rapid cycler and non-responsive to many of the most effective medications, making the illness more challenging to control. Nevertheless, he was encouraged by her, encouraged by who she was, and the kinds of choices she made. He shared his surprise and pleasure that Chloe continued to avoid drugs and alcohol, and was not involved in risky behavior like promiscuous sex or dangerous driving. This was unusual for a young person so severely affected by Bipolar Disorder. He told me then, and many other times, that Chloe's strong will was what kept her alive. He felt certain that as long as we persuaded her there was even a shred of hope, she would survive.

My journal reads: "Again. We begin again."

23
Early 2001

"The thing that is really hard, and really amazing, is giving up on being perfect and beginning the work of becoming yourself."
— Anna Quindlen

Throughout the month of January, Chloe slept, ate, and occasionally babysat. Although she did not re-sink to her lowest low, she was not getting better. She was no longer gaining weight, but was heavier than she felt comfortable. Her skin was a little clearer and her hair thickened up, but she looked sad and lost. She smiled and laughed only when with the children. Caring for them brought the only joy or light into her dark world.

One afternoon after watching Chloe and the children play with Jack, our miniature dachshund, Monica came up with what turned out to be a brilliant idea. She thought Chloe might like a pet of her own.

"Don't you think it would be good for Chloe to have something to take care of? Since she can't go to school right now, training a puppy would be a good project. It would give her something to do. Besides, when we're all gone Jack gets lonely. Another dog would be good for him, too."

My thirteen-year-old had developed a great plan. Hoping the responsibility for another life would help Chloe to value her own, we watched the newspaper for litters of dachshunds. In mid-February, we ran across an ad that sounded promising. I called the number and got directions to the home where the dogs were born. Chloe and I hopped in the car and drove across town, even more excited when we heard that there were three litters to choose from, twelve puppies.

When we got out of the car two full-grown dachshunds greeted us, and we knew we were at the right place. We went into the house and smiled at the set-up. One corner of the family room held two playpens, each containing a mother dog and her litter of pups. What remained of the third, older litter scampered about with two other adult dogs. Dachshunds were everywhere.

The owners encouraged us to look at all the puppies, pick them up, and get to know them as well as possible, but cautioned that one bunch was still too young to leave their mother. As Chloe picked up each little bundle, caressing their short, silky coats and nuzzling their tiny snouts, I thought she'd have a difficult time choosing. Then she picked up a tiny red female and we both knew she'd found the one.

From the still too-young litter, Chloe found a puppy whose miniature face bore distinct character, including a furrowed brow that made her look like a wise old woman. With warm brown eyes turned toward Chloe, this puppy wrinkled her forehead and poked her with a wet, pink nose. It looked as if she was doing the choosing. We were hooked. We painted her toenails to indicate she was taken, left a deposit, and went home, anticipating a phone call in two or three weeks when the puppy could leave her mother.

We were surprised when, just a few days later, the breeder called to say that the mother dog was refusing to nurse the puppies and they were eating solid food. We could pick up our little girl as soon as we'd like. Chloe wanted to go right there, right then, but we waited until Monica got home from school before we went to the pet store to get a kennel and puppy supplies, and then drove across town to pick up our new addition, Chloe's own pet.

Before we were halfway home, the puppy had become Molly, and we all thought she was perfect. Chloe was smitten. She loved Molly from the moment she laid eyes on her, and committed herself to that dog and the children she babysat. Through the rest of that month as well as the next, Chloe saw her doctor, rested a lot, and cared for Molly. For several years Molly was Chloe's link to living. When she thought she couldn't take any more mood swings or medication changes, she cooperated because Molly depended on her to be there.

When Chloe was miserable and stuck in bed, Molly snuggled under the covers with her. If Chloe felt better and

wanted to get outside, Molly was ready to romp. Molly was
Chloe's best friend. Aside from training and loving that puppy,
Chloe tended the little ones fairly regularly and occasionally saw
friends, but mostly she spent her time getting better. And she
painted.

Sometimes Chloe stayed up most of the night painting, no
longer working with pencils and pastels. Her artwork changed
dramatically, shifting from realistic figures and still-life
renditions to abstracts dominated by repetitive geometric
shapes. A different artist seemed to be at work. As she turned
nineteen, she was transforming again.

24
March 2001

*"I have myself an inner weight of woe
That God himself can scarcely bear."*
  — Theodore Roethke

When he turned sixteen in March 2001, Michael got a job at a local restaurant and seemed responsible and reliable. He never missed a shift and never went in late. Friends in the community often went there for dinner and shared laudatory comments about his manners, his behavior, and his ability to engage anybody in conversation. In addition to hearing how handsome Michael was, (six feet tall, with chiseled features, sandy blonde hair, bright green eyes, and an easy smile), we frequently heard about his charm. He was always polite and courteous. He smiled often and laughed easily, was fun to be around, the life of the party.

In many ways, he was like his dad. I felt proud of him, and happy that other people recognized and appreciated him. Nevertheless, I still heard occasional rumors about his partying and had a nagging feeling that Michael was experiencing great personal challenges. When I brought up the topic, he refused to talk and I did not push for more. Mark and I blindly figured that as long as he worked, went to school, and got good grades, everything must be fine.

In April, Chloe tried part-time work again, gaining a great deal of confidence at being able to do so. She was doing well enough that Mark and I felt safe traveling to San Francisco for a few days while my mom stayed with the children. When we returned, Chloe flew home with my mom to enjoy a week at her house in California. The two of them continued to share a close, loving connection, and Chloe was excited about the change of scenery. She always loved going to Gram's, and seemed to be having a good time when I talked to her on the phone. I detected some concern when I spoke with my mom, and wondered how Chloe was really feeling.

When I picked her up at the airport, Chloe's ill health was immediately apparent. Her mouth arched down in a frown, her glazed eyes were heavy-lidded, and furrows lined her brow. She looked sad and anxious. When I asked how she felt, she said she didn't feel good. She reverted to the frightened, childlike state we'd seen before. Her voice was that of a youngster. She asked others to do the simplest things for her, like getting a glass of juice or walking outside so she wouldn't be alone. She wanted me near at all times, expecting me to stay at her side until she fell asleep at night. She was unable to go to work, and asked me to call her manager. We called Dr. Kahil, who added another medication. Then came one of our all-time lows.

Exhausted and worn out by the constant care Chloe demanded, one night I simply told her no. The other children and Mark were already in bed and I told her I was going to bed, too. I would not sit up with her as I had been doing. I would not stay in her room until she fell asleep. I was tired and irritable and I wanted to go to sleep. She felt my indignation and commented on it.

"You don't want to take care of me any more."

"Chloe, that's not the deal. I'm tired. I'm sleepy. I just want to go to bed. You'll be fine. Either go to your room and work on a painting or read a book. Or, if you want, watch TV in the family room, but I'm not staying up any longer."

I went to bed.

An hour later, awakened by a shaft of light coming through my slowly opening door, I heard Chloe's voice: "Mommy, I did something really, really bad."

And she had.

From my journal on May 1, 2001: "I must begin in a new journal. I don't have the fortitude to continue in this one. My heart is too broken — is this volume a curse? I know it's not, but I do not want to use this book. Chloe took an overdose of Clonazapam today. Luckily she survived."

After I went to bed on that challenging night, Chloe fixated on my unwillingness to care for her, growing first angry, and then despondent. She assumed that I no longer wanted to be responsible for her care, and then decided that she did not want to live. She got her newly filled anti-anxiety prescription, took the whole thing, and then waited. As her anxiety began to abate, she realized she'd made a terrible mistake. That's when she came to my room.

When I heard her voice, I fully expected to see blood dripping from cut wrists, but was not surprised when she told me she'd taken the pills. Mark and I bundled her into the car and took her to the emergency room, knowing that we could get her there sooner than an ambulance could. I called the ER from my cell phone, explaining our situation.

By the time we arrived fifteen minutes later, Chloe was unable to hold up her head, much less stand. Mark parked at the curb, I dashed over to grab a wheelchair, and we pulled Chloe into it. We rushed her to the intake desk, handed the attending nurse the empty prescription bottle, and wheeled Chloe into triage, ahead of dozens of people waiting for care. The triage nurse asked Chloe a couple of questions, to which she could barely respond, and then another nurse aggressively approached her.

"What a selfish thing you've done. Can you not see what you're doing to your parents? Why in hell would you do this to yourself?"

Angered by her lack of professionalism, I was ready to give her a piece of my mind when Chloe raised her head only slightly and slowly but matter-of-factly told her, "I'm manic-depressive. I want to die."

The nurse blanched, gasped, then whispered, "I'm sorry," and whisked Chloe back to the treatment area. Mark and I remained at the intake desk to give vital information and wait until they called us back.

When we entered the curtained space where our daughter lay, the attending doctor introduced himself and told us that our quick action was fortunate, probably saving Chloe's life. They had pumped her stomach and filled it with charcoal to absorb whatever medication remained. She would stay there for several hours of close observation before moving to another room. Knowing she'd be there for a while, Mark and I stepped into the hall to develop a game plan for the day. We decided that he would go home to Michael and Monica while I stayed with Chloe.

When I returned to her bedside, Chloe was agitated. Enough of the drug had entered her bloodstream to render her a bit incoherent, but still quite anxious, and uninhibited. Like the times she experienced extreme mania, her language was foul and she was loud. Every few minutes the nurses came to check on her and asked questions to assess her condition. Each time she responded with belligerent, impatient answers.

"Chloe, can you hear me? How are you feeling?"

"Of course I can hear you. I'm not deaf. I'm suicidal. And in case you're wondering, most suicidal people don't feel real good."

With each round of questions, she became more rude and disrespectful. Slurring her words and raising her voice, she screamed, "How the fuck do you think I'm doing? I want to die and nobody will let me. I'm not doing too great. Why don't you assholes just leave me alone?"

Appalled and embarrassed, I tried to settle her down. "Chloe, stop talking like that and lower your voice. These people are doing their jobs. They're doing their best to help you and I want you to stop treating them like crap."

Then she directed her anger at me. "Fuck you. I don't care what you want. You have no idea how I feel or what's best for me. What do you care anyway? Besides, what makes you think they're doing their best for me? You're my mother and you don't even want to take care of me."

Then she decided she wanted to go home. Her whole affect changed. Her face, tight and grimacing as she spat out her words, softened. Her eyes welled with tears, her lips trembled, and her chin quivered. "I'm sorry, Mommy. I want to go home. I won't do it again. I promise. Please, just take me home."

It surprises me even now that on that night Chloe honestly thought she could come so close to taking her own life, and then simply go home a few hours later. The gravity of the situation failed to register with her.

Interestingly, at about the same time, the hospital staff contacted Dr. Kahil to inform him of her suicide attempt.

Knowing that in the past I had worked hard to keep Chloe out of the psychiatric hospital, he waived the usual seventy-two-hour stay, telling the nurses that I knew best and he would leave the decision to me. Shortly after talking to him, one of the nurses caring for Chloe came into the treatment area and shared what he had said.

I couldn't do it. I could not be responsible for keeping her alive. I needed a break. I asked the staff to admit her to the psychiatric hospital across the street. When she heard my decision, she exploded with anger. Even now, years later, I think that was my most challenging moment with Chloe.

She screamed, "Leave me alone you fucking bitch. I hate you. You did this to me. It's your fault I'm here. You don't want to fucking take care of me, so leave. I don't want you near me. I hate you. Leave!"

Chloe had never spewed that kind of venom at me, and I was both frightened and taken aback. I did not know this person. She refused to look at or listen to me.

"Chloe, listen to me."

"Fuck you. No. No. No. I will not listen to you. Leave. Leave me. That's what you want to do, you bitch. So leave."

Every time I tried to talk she shouted strings of obscenities over my voice and wouldn't stop until I was out of her sight. Shaken to the core, I stood behind a curtain in the emergency room, gasping for breath and struggling to maintain my composure. The staff wisely gave me a few minutes before encouraging me to go home. I could not. Despite the fact that she wanted me to leave, I knew Chloe wasn't herself and I didn't want her to feel abandoned. When I re-entered the treatment area she bombarded me with another verbal assault.

"I love you, Chloe, and I want to help you feel better. If you need me, I'll be just around the corner."

"I don't want you here and I don't want you just around the corner." Then to the nurses, "Make her leave." Then back to me, "Get out of here. Go. Leave. Leave me."

I walked into the hall and called Mark. Sobbing, I told him what was going on. "I'm sorry Mark, but I can't bring her home. I can't do it any more. I can't take care of her this way. Not right now. Please come back. Talk to her, Mark. She'll listen to you."

In less than thirty minutes, Mark was at Chloe's bedside.

"Daddy, please take me home. I feel better and won't try anything. I was mad at Mom, but I'm not mad anymore. I'm not going to do anything bad. I want to go home."

"Honey, you have to stay in the hospital. You're not well and Mom and I need help to take care of you. We can't keep you safe. The doctors and nurses can do that."

"I don't want to be in the hospital," she screamed. "You're taking Mom's side. I hate her. She just doesn't want to take care of me any more. She won't have to. I'll take care of myself. You're both wrong. I'm fine. LET ME COME HOME." Looking at me, she shouted, "I hate you. You act like you love me, but you don't. This is your fault. You're the reason I'm here. I hate you."

Wisely, Mark realized we were doing no good and that my presence perpetuated, even exacerbated, her angry ranting. I'd been in the emergency room for six hours when I told Chloe I loved her and walked away, chased down the hall by a litany of foul, furious words.

Chloe went to the psychiatric hospital later that day and I didn't see her for two more. I called her workplace, explaining that she was in the hospital, and I arranged to have her babysitting responsibilities covered. I got her things together in a paper bag, and sent them with Mark during visiting hour the next evening. I could not convince myself to go see her until a little time had passed. By the time I did, she was more in control and feeling remorseful for what she had said and done. Both of us in a clearer state of mind, and we began to heal.

One of the greatest curses of Bipolar Disorder is the guilt and anxiety its victims feel in the aftermath of behavior that is essentially out of their control. I know now, and I knew then, that Chloe, in a balanced and well state, would never have behaved or spoken the way she did. I knew it was her illness, and not her true self, that motivated the events. Nevertheless, she did not feel confident about what I believed, and we had to talk about it repeatedly before she was sure that we understood each another.

Chloe stayed in the hospital for nearly a week during which time a new doctor monitored her very closely, reviewed the previous two years of treatment, and made significant medication changes. In addition to those developments, I decided she could not come home until we had a family appointment with Maria. This episode shook us up and I had some thoughts and emotions to sort and share.

The day after Chloe came home from the hospital all five of us went to Maria's office. We settled into her small space so that everyone could see one another. A palpable tension permeated the room, as if we held powerfully charged words that would electrify the air if we let them out.

Maria began, "Chloe, Why don't you tell us what happened before your parents took you to the hospital last week."

She answered quite matter-of-factly, "I felt like my mom didn't want to take care of me any more and I didn't think I could take care of myself, so I wanted to die. After I took the pills, I knew I shouldn't have. I knew I didn't want to die. I really wanted to live, even if I had to live with Bipolar."

What a huge realization. I was glad that Chloe reached what seemed to be a new plateau in her recovery. Maria then opened the floor to the rest of us, beginning with Monica.

"I'm glad Chloe's better. I was mad that she took the pills, but I'm not mad now. I'm glad she doesn't want to die. I want her to be like she used to be."

Michael slumped in his chair and, obviously unhappy about being there, crossed his arms over his chest and said, "I don't have anything to say. This is Chloe's deal, not mine. I don't think it's any of my business. I don't even want to be here."

Maria pressed, "But how do you feel about Chloe's illness and its effects on your family? How do you feel about what happened last week, Michael? This is your opportunity to ask questions and get answers."

"She's better. I don't need to know anything else."

And that was that. My concern for his well-being grew.

Mark voiced his concerns as if he was at a business meeting. He worked hard to keep his emotions in check, and this was another example of that.

"Well, let's see," he began, "I guess I want some assurances from Chloe that this won't happen again. I want her to tell us when she's feeling worse so we can help her before it gets to this point. And," looking Chloe right in the eye, "I never want you to treat your mom that way again."

Chloe assured us that she could comply with those wishes and apologized again, for how she had treated me.

Then it was my turn.

I felt like an unknotted helium balloon released from a firm grip. The words flew out of my mouth as if time might expire before I said all that I needed to say. "I feel so guilty for not taking better care of you, Chloe, for allowing your illness to get to the point that you felt like you had to take the pills. But I want you to know, I want all of you to know, that I can't be responsible for keeping Chloe alive. I just cannot do it, and I am so afraid that if she tries to kill herself again, and she succeeds, the rest of you will blame me. I don't want it to be my responsibility. I don't want it to be my fault. This is not my fault."

My tears flowed as I continued, "Chloe, I love you so much, and I want you to be well, but I can't make you well. I kept thinking I could. I kept thinking it was my job to keep you alive. When you took those pills, I realized how inadequate I am. I can't keep you alive. You have the power to take your own life, and if you're determined to do that, I'm helpless. I can't stop you. So I'm telling you, I'll do everything I can to help you get better, but I cannot, I will not, be held responsible for your death."

That May 2001 day was a turning point. I no longer made it my responsibility to keep Chloe alive. It was as if, up until that time, I had considered myself godlike, with power to give and take life. When I admitted my helplessness in the situation, things began to change. I'd spent the previous two years absorbed by Chloe and her illness. Even though I still cared for the rest of my family and mothered my other two children, for those two years Chloe was my primary focus and everybody knew it. Our lives were terribly askew, and the time had come to correct that. Again, this chaotic, sometimes catastrophic illness taught me to appreciate another elemental truth: Balance. Balance is necessary in all things.

Balance is vital to well-being.

I had to find balance within myself, and then allow that balance to guide my actions to create equilibrium in our family life. My actions could then cause ripples of change in those around me and balance would begin to perpetuate itself.

Perhaps Chloe would find balance in mood and thought that would allow her to find her place in this world.

From my journal: "As foolish as this sounds, I just realized something vastly important. We can simultaneously experience great highs and lows. Albert Einstein once said, 'In the middle of difficulty lies opportunity.' I want to take advantage of every opportunity afforded me. I want to learn what these highs and lows can teach. I want to embrace the challenge and grow. I must not let life's challenges drag me into the abyss and prevent my enjoying its blessings. The blessings are there. They are always there."

25
June 2001

"To create is always to learn, to begin over, to begin at zero."
  — Matthew Fox

From the moment I confessed my inadequacies in Maria's office, Chloe and I had a different relationship. It developed beyond mother and child and became more respectful, more mature. The next several months passed with an increasing level of comfort and ease between us. A sense of calm enveloped our family and we responded less viscerally when Chloe experienced ups or downs, or all-arounds. We learned to take things in stride and not panic. I suppose we finally began to accept her diagnosis and the permanence of her illness. We stopped chasing the cure and yearning for what used to be. We looked forward, toward what life could become, and embraced blessings that always were. What relief.

It was also a relief to Chloe that Mark and I accepted her, illness and all, as whole and right. We no longer wanted to "fix" her. We were learning to accept the mood swings and unusual responses to things as simply a part of who she was. We both hoped that she could develop skills and strategies to live with the Bipolar and be as content as possible. Most of all, we knew without a doubt that we loved her unconditionally, regardless of what she said or what she did.

She felt that all-encompassing acceptance. Together we moved into a different arena, making goals for ongoing wellness and future success built around her brilliance and creativity. It became our goal to keep her stable enough to do what she desired rather than to eradicate the Bipolar Disorder and return to old ideas of what she ought to be and what she ought to do. We grew and moved on.

Chloe went back to work part-time and the rest of us fell into a less frenetic summer routine. The children were out of school and we planned fun vacations, including a week at the beach and a long weekend at a nearby resort. We spent a lot of time together as a family, yet each of us pursued individual interests and activities. June was, for the first time in many months, close to normal. Except that it marked the beginning of Michael's Bipolar experience, even though I seemed to be the only one who knew that.

Throughout the preceding spring, Michael attended school, worked three of four nights a week, and hung out with his friends. Although several times I suspected he was drinking to excess, I did not follow up on my suspicions. I told myself I was overreacting, that he was a great kid. We kept hearing good things about him, so I tried not to worry. Sadly, my suspicions were correct, and by the time school was out, we had repeatedly disciplined him for drinking and smoking marijuana.

I thought we were dealing with more than typical teenage experimentation. I also knew that I had less tolerance than most people because of my background. I second-guessed myself and failed to trust my gut instincts. Soon I could no longer do that. Michael's substance abuse mushroomed. I caught him in several lies and found him seriously drunk more than once. I also discovered marijuana paraphernalia and baggies containing small amounts of pot in his laundry, his bedroom, and the car. My extreme reactions grew from emotions firmly rooted in my own childhood.

My father was an aggressive and often violent alcoholic, and one of my brothers, beginning at age thirteen, walked that same difficult path. I knew what addict behaviors looked like. I was familiar with the patterns of blame and excuses, and felt frightened by the possibility that I could live that nightmare again. I did not want to do that. Long ago, I promised myself that I would never again live with an alcoholic or an addict, and I had no patience or tolerance for it. Of course, I never fathomed that one of my children would become one.

I came down hard. I yelled, pleaded, begged, and accused. I turned into a police officer, checking his backpack, going through his room, closely monitoring his whereabouts and his comings and goings. Our relationship, which had always been warm, loving, and accepting, became adversarial. It was Michael against me, but I could not see that. I insisted I was doing what parents of teens should do when they suspect drug abuse. I was absolute in my righteous indignation. My fears grew every time I found more evidence of drug and alcohol use, and I vented those fears on Mark who struggled to determine the difference between experimentation and chronic abuse. He, too, feared for our son.

It was with great concern and a lot of anger that we entered the arena of drug and alcohol abuse that accompanies Juvenile Onset Bipolar Disorder an estimated eighty percent of the time. In retrospect, I don't know why I wasn't more compassionate and accepting. From the time Chloe and I first encountered the mental health scene, every new caregiver asked about a history of drug and alcohol abuse and promiscuity. Doctors and nurses repeatedly told me I was lucky since they rarely saw children as sick as Chloe who had not experimented with substances or acted out sexually. I'd learned to let go and accept in regards to Chloe's health, but this topic was a real trigger for me. I was far from that kind of acceptance when it came to Michael and his behaviors. I am such a slow learner.

From my journal on June 10, 2001: "Am I running fearfully in circles in the dark, wearing a rut so deep in the ground that I'll never escape?"

I called Dr. Sander and Dr. Kahil to get recommendations for counselors and psychologists specializing in teens with substance-abuse issues. I finally decided on one highly recommended doctor and made an appointment. Michael was not happy about going and declared his intention to be uncooperative. He didn't deny smoking weed and drinking, but insisted it was not abuse, it was use. He asserted that his use was different from most of his friends', but refused to elaborate. Mark and I accompanied him to his first appointment and the doctor thought issues existed that we could resolve together. We made a series of follow-up appointments.

From my journal on June 11, 2001: "God wisely divided time into twenty-four-hour increments and made us diurnal creatures, forcing us to stop our senseless activity and begin anew when the sun comes up. His infinite wisdom is reflected in everything if we take time to notice it. There it is again—time. Use it wisely. Appreciate it. Know that it heals all wounds if we move with it and refuse to be stuck in one spot. It's a challenge, it's a gift."

Because Mark's work left him unable to get away every week, Michael and I continued to see the psychologist together. Michael and the doctor were together for most of each session, and I joined them for the last few minutes. I shared my concerns about not only the substance abuse, but also the possibility that Michael could have Bipolar Disorder, since his older sister did.

The doctor, who seemed well versed in the language of substance abuse, but less informed on the topic of chronic mental illness, didn't think that was evident, but cautioned us to be aware of the possibility. He also told me to lower my expectations regarding the outcome of our sessions. He said the situation was not as bad as I perceived it to be. This should have been a red flag for me, but it wasn't. We saw him a few more times.

The last session with the psychologist stands out as one of the greatest failings of a medical practitioner in our experience. Michael spent a few minutes with the doctor before I went in. The doctor asked Michael to tell me how he perceived his marijuana and alcohol use.

"I don't have a problem. I know you and Dad think I do, but I don't. I only use when I want to. I don't use when I don't feel like it, even if other people are using. I'm not addicted. I choose when I get high. It's not affecting my grades or work, so I don't see why you're making such a big deal out of it. It's my choice, my decision. No matter how often you bring me here, I'm not gonna stop."

Then the doctor turned to me.

"How do you feel about that?"

Against my own will, I began to cry.

"I'm so scared for you Michael. I watched my dad and my brother make these same choices. I've heard these exact words and I'm afraid. If you can stop whenever you want, then please stop, for me. I'm afraid you could have Bipolar Disorder, and if you do, we'll never get proper care as long as you're using pot and alcohol. It's not safe for you to do these things. I just want you to stop."

Michael had no response, but the doctor did.

"Mrs. McLaughlin, you have to accept the fact that this is your problem, not Michael's. You have a great kid here. He follows most of your rules, he gets good grades, he's responsible at work, and other adults like and respect him. What you have is an ordinary teenage boy—no, an extraordinary young man— who is experimenting. Stop worrying. He'll be fine. You've got to let it go."

In front of Michael, a medical professional, an expert, just told me if there was a problem, that problem was mine. I felt like I'd been taken out at the knees. I was at a complete and total loss. My son had just received permission to continue his substance abuse and I did not have a leg to stand on. We never went back.

26
August-December 2001

"The bravest are surely those who have the clearest vision of what is before them, glory and danger alike, and yet notwithstanding go out to meet it."
— Thucydides

In August 2001, thirteen-year-old Monica and sixteen-year-old Michael started back to school, followed a week later by Chloe, who was now nineteen. She took twelve units against her doctor's advice, wanting to jump back into school. She needed to participate in academia, to succeed again in the arena by which she defined herself. She needed to move into her own future. She did so boldly and confidently, making great progress in the face of great adversity.

Despite the fact that doing too much might cause a serious relapse, Chloe continued to work a shift or two a week. Making even a small amount of spending money made her feel less dependent and more responsible. She bravely explained her illness to her immediate supervisor, cautioning her that a period of instability could cause her to miss work. If she got quite ill, she would need a leave of absence.

They worked out an agreement wherein Chloe would call one of several people to cover her shift if that became necessary. Then her supervisor did something very unusual. She told Chloe about her own chronic health problem and decade-long struggle to get back into the work force. She commended Chloe on her brave openness. Chloe worked through the semester, taking a leave when she enrolled in classes that were more difficult in the spring.

Chloe also took on complete responsibility for her own medical care. She no longer relied on me to remind her to take her meds or phone in refills when she ran low. She went to the pharmacy herself, and asked questions about side effects and contraindications since she took so many prescriptions. She made her own appointments and, although she continued to seek my opinion and support, she made her own treatment decisions. She gained confidence and began to project a future in which she could have the kind of life she sought.

Equally encouraging was the manner in which she tackled other facets of her life. She continued to see Maria, developing strategies and techniques to improve her communication and social skills when she was not feeling well. She talked to me about those strategies, and a time or two asked me to role-play with her to put them to the test. Most significantly, she developed the ability to analyze herself and her responses, and to realize when those responses were inappropriate. She was on the fast track toward self-improvement.

With increasing confidence, Chloe also made efforts to develop her interests, social contacts, intellect, and physical health. When she knew we would be buying holiday and birthday gifts, she asked for art supplies so she could continue to draw, paint, and sketch. She also picked up poetry and literature books from a local used bookstore and read voraciously. She was seeing more of her friends, too, choosing times and places that were compatible with her needs. She took care not to challenge her still-fragile health.

With Maria's help, Chloe evaluated her mental status over the preceding two years and identified trends and triggers. She figured out what to expect at different times of the year and learned to recognize changes in her body and in her mind when her health took a turn for the worse. She was learning to accept and live with the illness. She was making the best of it—choosing the high road.

From my journal on September 2001: "For every life experience, we choose a fork in the road. We may choose the high road or we may choose the low road, but we most certainly do choose."

The warmth of late summer melted into fall. Chloe continued to hold her own, babysitting and excelling at school. Michael, however, was having trouble, and we feared that he was getting more deeply involved in the party scene. We talked to him, but didn't take much action. Still reeling from our last visit to the psychologist several weeks earlier, I didn't know what to do.

As the semester progressed, Michael became more difficult to get out of bed in the morning. For most kids, this is not unusual, but Michael had gotten up by himself since first grade. We'd never had this problem, even in early adolescence when it's most common. I attributed it to working too many shifts and suggested he stick to weekends, but his boss was short-handed and needed him through the week. Not wanting to force the issue, I made it clear that he'd have to quit working altogether if his grades suffered.

We spent Thanksgiving week in California, visiting family, and staying and playing at Disneyland. It was pure fun and one of the first trips Chloe was able to take without falling apart afterward. Michael and Monica had a wonderful time too, as the three of them began to rebuild their strained and sometimes difficult relationships. Happily, Michael seemed like himself. There were no drugs or alcohol, no upsetting incidents to take away from the joy. We returned home feeling rejuvenated and reconnected. It was a very good time.

A couple weeks later, in the early morning of a cool, fall Saturday, one of Mark's nieces called. Living in the Midwest, she had her hands full with three little girls and an in-home daycare business. We often talked about the children and enjoyed a warm relationship. This time, the conversation was quite different as she told me one of her daughters dad been diagnosed with Juvenile Onset Bipolar Disorder.

She wanted to know more about her grandmother, since she was already making the familial connections I had made months earlier. We talked for a long time, comparing notes, medical information, and reading material. We realized that there were probably other cases of Bipolar Disorder, concealed or undiagnosed, in our extended family.

That conversation was bittersweet. We were happy to have a trusted family member with whom we could share our experiences. We were sad that other loved ones were living through the challenges.

When I attended Michael's parent-teacher conferences at the end of the semester it was obvious we had a big problem. Not only had every grade dropped, but also for the first time in his life, teachers commented negatively on his attitude, effort, and citizenship. It was like listening to a report about a different child, and that's how teachers who taught him the previous year felt. His poor showing was disappointing and surprising. Mark and I talked about the change and then talked to Michael. I brought up the subject of alcohol and marijuana use, which he, of course, adamantly denied being factors in the academic decline. He admitted that he was not doing his homework or trying as hard as usual, then promised second semester would be different.

Chloe's health improved. In December, she worked more shifts and spent a lot of time with Michael and Monica. Even a week's worth of out-of-town company failed to disturb the balance she had achieved. She still cycled frequently, but her medications and determination kept her balanced enough to function better than she had in a long time. We felt encouraged that Chloe could have a wonderful, full life. For her, 2001 ended on the high road and we had hopes of continuing that trend.

27
Early 2002

"No excellent soul is exempt from a mixture of madness."
— Aristotle

In January 2002, Chloe began the spring semester carrying twelve units. She babysat two or three times a week and was only seeing Maria and Dr. Kahil once a month. She spent a lot of time with Eric, a friend she had met during the fall semester, and began parking at his house, then walking to class from there. He soon became one of her closest friends and she was thrilled to have the camaraderie again. They studied together during the week, hung out and played with Molly on the weekends, and sometimes dated one another's friends. It was a fun, healthy relationship, and we were happy she was getting out more. We were sure it was a good sign.

Then she came home with the news that she had gone back to the restaurant where she used to hostess and took on a part-time position. I was surprised since she hadn't mentioned adding work back into her schedule. I felt concern, but didn't want to throw a spin on what might be another step toward regaining her health. About the same time, she began dating a young man with whom she quickly became quite serious. They spent all of their free time together or on the phone. It seemed like too much, too fast, but I'd begun dating Mark when I was seventeen, and knew right away that he was the one for me. My experience told me it could happen. My gut told me to beware.

After only a few weeks of this heightened routine, Chloe's health began to crumble. She went back to weekly visits with both Dr. Kahil and Maria, and dropped six units to reduce the pressure she felt at school. One day she called me while on a break at work and told me she didn't feel good. We talked for a few minutes, she settled down, and went back to her shift.

In less than an hour, the phone rang again. When I answered there was no response, but caller ID told me it was Chloe. I heard crying and gasping, but she did not speak.

"Chloe, what's the matter? Where are you?"

No response.

"Are you still at work? What happened? Tell me what's wrong."

After what felt like a very long time, she was able to answer when I again asked what was happening, and where she was.

"I'm...in...the parking lot...behind...the restaurant."

"I'll be right there."

Shortly after our first conversation she felt overwhelmed by anxiety, then panicked and left the dining room without telling anyone. When she got to her car, she realized she was shaking too much to drive and dissolved into uncontrollable tears. I drove to the parking lot behind the restaurant and found my daughter sitting on the curb outside the kitchen, shirt untucked, sobbing, rocking back and forth, and chain-smoking. Mascara ran down her cheeks, her shoes were off, and her hair looked like she had clenched it in her fists and pulled. She brought a cigarette to and from her mouth in stiff, shaky movements, fingers white and hyper-extended from tension.

Between the smoking and the crying, I'm not sure how any oxygen got to her brain. I sat next to her on the curb and rubbed her back until she settled down.

"Tell me what happened."

She really didn't know and might not have been able to articulate it if she did. I went inside and told her manager that she'd gotten sick and called me, and that I was taking her home. She must have wanted greater explanation, and it must have seemed strange for a grown woman's mom to come in as if she was a child leaving school early. She was kind and compassionate, asking Chloe to call when she felt better. It was good to receive acceptance and concern from someone who had every right to be upset.

I drove Chloe home, where she took her anti-anxiety medication. When she finally fell asleep, Michael accompanied me back to the restaurant to retrieve her car. Chloe slept for the rest of the evening and through the night, but the meltdown left her groggy and blue for several days. It was a long time before we saw a healthier Chloe emerge again.

For weeks, she endured the discomfort of combined mania and depression. This "mixed state" persisted, despite schedule changes, medication adjustments, and frequent doctor visits. I knew this was the most difficult mood state to control, and probably the most dangerous.

In *Night Falls Fast*, author Kay Redfield Jamison says: "Behavior and moods during these periods tends to be volatile and erratic. Any combination of symptoms is possible, but the one most virulent for suicide is the mix of depressive mood, morbid thinking, and a 'wired,' agitated level of energy. Paranoia, extreme irascibility, fitful sleep, heavy drinking, and physical lashing out not uncommonly go along with this particular variant of a mixed state. It is singularly and dangerously uncomfortable. Excess energy produces a kind of unhinging agitation, and 'almost terrible energy,' as poet Anne Sexton put it."

Dr. Kahil and Maria worked to gain control over Chloe's current state, but her brain chemistry and electrical functions seemed determined to resist that control. Mark and I feared that hospitalization was just around the corner, but we maintained hope that Chloe would persist and improve. She, of course, did not want to drop her remaining classes. It was so important to finish the semester and feel like a success in at least one arena.

As her health continued to be fragile, Chloe and her boyfriend were at the house all the time. He wanted to help, but didn't know what to do. A nice young man who cared a lot, he asked questions about her illness, treatment, and prognosis. He slept on the floor next to her bed when she was too distraught to be alone. He stayed awake with her when mania prevented sleep. He drove her to and from class on those rare times she was able to make it, and supported her even though her moods and attitudes made that support difficult. I felt relieved that Chloe could trust someone other than me when she felt poorly. That alone was progress.

Because she could not tolerate the way she felt or the things she thought, Chloe had a hard time with the rest of us. When a person is struggling in a mixed state, "moody" and "difficult to get along with" do not even come close to describing the situation. She was increasingly contentious and her boyfriend joined her in that mood. They argued more often than not, each blaming the other at every juncture. By semester's end, her health had badly eroded and her relationship had done the same. She finished classes, broke up with her beau, and agreed to go into the hospital. However, that hospital stay was very short.

Chloe moved from a mixed state to extreme mania. Less than twenty-four hours after her admission into the hospital, her mood became unnaturally elevated and her outlook ebulliently optimistic. Delusions of grandeur were hard at work. In just a few days, she convinced the hospital staff that she was well and balanced, and called me from the lobby, saying she'd already checked herself out and needed a ride home. I did not think she was well enough to come home yet, but she assured me she was fine and said she was better off at home because the psych techs were hitting on her and flirting with her. When she got a phone call from one of those techs on the way home, I knew not all was well. However, I had neither the right nor the power to make her stay in the hospital.

I'd picked her up from the hospital just past noon, and by evening Chloe was dressed up, made up, and heading out for a night on the town. I was worried. She checked in by telephone and came home before midnight. Once she was safely home, I turned off my light and tried to go to sleep. Keyed up after worrying all evening, I could not. I got up and went into her bedroom.

She was gone.

She had left a note:

"Mom-
Gone to Gram's. Don't worry. Call you when I get there.
Love,
Chloe."

The only problem—Gram lived 450 miles away.

Fear gripped me. Envisioning a manic Chloe, flying down the dark highway with little concern for safety, I ran back to our bedroom and woke Mark. All of the horrible, possible outcomes played out in my mind. I knew these periods of grandiosity were brief interludes before extreme anxiety and agitation set in. I worried that the shift would happen quickly and Chloe would be suicidal or psychotic since both had happened in the past. My stomach knotted and my heart pounded. Rushing adrenaline guaranteed a wakeful night during which I had to bridle my fear and imagination, and rely on hope and faith.

Mark and I tried to reach Chloe on her cell phone, but she seemed to be following our rule and didn't answer while driving. We briefly discussed calling the sheriff or highway patrol, but feared an approach of sirens and lights could be her undoing. Then I called my mom in California and filled her in, so she'd be ready for Chloe's impromptu arrival. After that, I called Chloe's friends to get a handle on what had happened during the evening.

When she arrived far sooner than she should have, Chloe called from my mom's as if nothing were out of the ordinary. I told her to get some sleep while Gram was at work, and call me when she woke up. I called Dr. Kahil and Maria, and they both insisted that Chloe was not safe and that I needed to get her home as soon as possible. When my mom got to work, she called me and we decided that she would drive Chloe home the next day and then fly back to California.

As the hours passed, several of Chloe's friends returned my calls, expressing concern over her odd behavior. I heard the same thing repeatedly. She was not her usual self. She was using foul and suggestive language, laughing too hard, talking too quickly, behaving provocatively, and generally coming on too strong and too loud. They described a textbook case of mania, confirming my suspicions and her doctor's fears.

The following evening Mom and Chloe arrived at the house, totally wiped out. Chloe's mania had already shifted gears and she was exhausted despite having slept the entire ride home. Mom drove straight through and worried herself into her own state of exhaustion. I was relieved we'd made it through a potentially dangerous incident with no harm done. Chloe saw Dr. Kahil the next day. Fortunately, even she agreed that her behavior was unacceptable, but commented, "I'm still ticked off that you didn't let me enjoy a California vacation after I went through all the effort to get there so quickly."

I had to laugh. I could see Chloe and the long-haul drivers soaring across the desert at break-neck speed. At least we could finally have a sense of humor about the unusual experiences spawned by her illness.

Chloe's mood had quickly shifted from a mixed state to mania. She had difficulty explaining the sensations, and I couldn't accurately recount or describe what led to the shift. I still knew too little about the onset of mania, and searched the internet for more information. That is when I came across a website created anonymously by a young woman with Bipolar Disorder. She offered the following description of the onset of her mania, which I found informative and helpful:

"My first sign of mania is anger. I am by nature a person with absolutely no temper—unless I am manic. When I feel myself getting angry about things I cannot control, and getting angry at people, I know I might be getting manic.

"After that, another symptom is having a constant smile on my face that I can't wipe off. The smile hurts. It's exhausting. I also notice right away that I hear voices and see things when I'm trying to fall asleep. Then I start getting ideas of things I need to do—learn how to bake things, reorganize everything in my house, call all of my friends, (but the minute I have them on the phone I'm too agitated to concentrate on one thing).

"All those, for me, are the very first stage. Next, my mind switches from wondering whether I might be getting manic, and being concerned about it, to knowing I am getting manic, denying to myself that anyone can help. Then I go inside myself—I see things, hear things, have huge conspiracy theories, and I can't tell anyone. I have to hide from cameras on lampposts and traffic lights. Everything I see is symbolic, a puzzle for me to put together.

"Next, I stop sleeping completely. I can't eat. I need constant noise, two or three sources at once, or all I can hear is silence and it scares the hell out of me. I try to have conversations with people—while hiding all I suspect—and I can't stay on one subject. People get tired of talking to me because my speech is uninterrupted. I can't make myself stop to let them respond. Then, the television starts talking to me. I start collecting things that seem to have significance—used Band-Aids, newspaper articles, twigs.

"Finally, I become terrified of myself, terrified of people who love me, terrified to be found out and caught and locked up—I know when I get hospitalized that all this important knowledge that's central to my survival will be erased. My mind will be wiped clear. I'll have another camera implanted under my skin, and I'll never again have a moment alone. I talk to strangers, pleading with them about things like going to heaven and avoiding FBI surrounding tactics. My driving is dangerous. I can't be bothered with traffic lights. I get hurt. I get hit on the head, cuts, bruises—I get hurt because I can't pay attention to how my body feels, I'm trying to save my mind.

"Usually about this time, I get hospitalized. I'm somewhere and the police come. The whole process can happen in three or four days, or it can stretch out to a month."

This candid and articulate account of a frightening and embarrassing result of mental illness provided me with insight and compassion as we continued to learn more about living with chronic illness, Bipolar Disorder in particular, and the evolutionary effect it had on each of us.

28

Early spring 2002

"I do not love him because he is good, but because he is my child."
— Rabindranath Tagore

As surprised as my mom was to receive our late-night phone call and then Chloe on her doorstep, she was even more stunned by Michael's appearance when she brought Chloe home. Gaunt physique and dark-rimmed, bloodshot eyes revealed at least a portion of what his last few months had been like, and she was unprepared for the radical change. Although I had been very open with her about Chloe's situation, I had not shared details of Michael's recent challenges or my nagging suspicions.

Looking back, I was ashamed of Michael's drug use and ashamed of myself for not being able to prevent it. Most profoundly, dealing with issues of drugs and alcohol again brought back myriad suppressed and unpleasant memories from my childhood, and I was ashamed of the unkind thoughts, comments, and actions I'd directed toward my parents when I was younger.

As I grew up my mom, my siblings, and I blamed my dad's drinking for every problem within the family. As my brother embarked on that same path behind my father, we shifted some of the blame to him. In turn, I blamed both of my parents for my brother's illegal and anti-social behaviors. I judged them harshly and often. As is always the case when one fails to approach life's big learning opportunities with love and acceptance, I found myself reliving the same issues, embroiled in the same snares my parents struggled against so many years ago. Those snares bound and gagged me, disallowing the acceptance and honesty I would later develop.

At the time, Mark and I could not agree on how to deal with Michael, and the already loaded topic took on an additional emotional charge. It almost felt dangerous to discuss Michael's drug and alcohol use with anyone else. Knowing our family patterns and dynamics so well, I also feared my mom's judgment of Michael and wanted to protect him, as I still do when people hear about his history of substance abuse. I want others to adore him as I do. He is precious.

From the moment I held a newborn Michael in my arms, I idolized him. I remember the warm, musty smell and soft texture of his downy, blonde hair. I was enthralled with his huge blue eyes, that later changed to the same green as mine. Even as a baby, his broad shoulders and strong build fascinated me. Unlike newborn Chloe, he was content. He smiled often and was easily soothed. He slept well and entertained himself a long time before wanting to be picked up. He was a much easier infant, thank goodness.

Michael had dozens of respiratory infections his first five years, leading to tests for serious illnesses including Cystic Fibrosis and AIDS. When the tests came back negative, his doctors determined that his body developed an inappropriate immune response to viruses, almost as if he was allergic to them. This overreaction led to respiratory infections. They predicted, and rightly so, that as he matured the condition would subside. By age six, he was as healthy and happy, living with asthma as a residual reminder of his early health issues.

Michael spent his childhood generously giving of himself. He was kind and empathic toward others, deeply feeling what others felt. He smiled and laughed often, easily connecting with others. We joked that he could make friends in the grocery store line. His natural gregariousness and classic little-boy good looks made him easy to like. He sailed through elementary school and junior high as one of the brightest boys in his class. He always got good grades, was student council president, and the girls loved him. His teachers praised him, parents of his friends enjoyed having him around, and his dad, sisters, and I thought he was nearly perfect. The phone rang for him more than the rest of us combined. He was charming. Prophetically, two years earlier a teacher predicted, "Michael's charm will be his downfall." It was.

With the demands of Chloe's care overwhelming us, and the upbraiding I'd received from Michael's psychologist dogging me, I failed to act on additional warning signs that my son was in trouble. I hoped and prayed that his situation would improve on it's own since I didn't know what to do next. I felt stretched too thin and regretted spending too little one-on-one time with Monica and Michael, but did not yet have the tools to correct that. We did our best to cope. Michael was doing his best to cope, too, but the past several weeks indicated that his drug and alcohol use were increasing. The first sign came in the form of a phone call early one evening.

Michael had not come home from school and I began to worry. When the phone rang and caller I.D. told me it was a friend of his, I grabbed the phone with relief. It was Michael. He was at Colin's house and wanted to know if he could spend the night because a bunch of guys were playing video games. My heart jumped into my throat and my voice stuck there with it. Michael sounded unlike himself, speaking thickly and slurring his words. I felt like I was talking to my dad on the phone. I told him no, Mark and I would be pick him up in a few minutes, so he should get his things together. He tried to argue with me but was so wasted he couldn't make his mouth work. I got off the phone and told Mark.

When we got to Colin's house, Michael staggered out the front door and down the driveway, remaining upright by teetering against the cars parked there. A friend of his followed him to our car.

"I'm so glad you came to get Michael. He's so messed up, everybody's worried about him." Then she told me that she was worried about Michael in general.

"This is happening more and more. He gets totally wasted and out of control. I'm afraid he's going to get hurt. Normally, I wouldn't say anything, but I think something's wrong. I'm not the only one who's tried to talk to him, but Michael won't listen to any of us."

There it was. The truth told by an innocent, concerned friend. I was no longer jumping to conclusions or imagining that things were worse than they actually were.

Since it was clear that any kind of dialogue was impossible, we took Michael home and told him to go to bed, deciding to talk to him in the morning. Then Mark and I talked. I was terribly concerned, but Mark still thought Michael was on the extreme edge, but within the bounds of normal teenage behavior. I wanted to seek counseling or get some help, and Mark thought we should talk to Michael, lay down more stringent ground rules, and mete out the necessary consequences. I reluctantly agreed.

The next morning we three sat down and talked about the incident. Initially Michael tried to con us, "I wasn't that far gone, and besides, I only got so wasted because Colin put 'bud' in the brownies and didn't tell me. He thought it was funny. What an idiot. I won't hang out there any time soon."

When we didn't buy the snow job, and told him as much, Michael grew defensive and argumentative.

"You guys don't know what you're talking about. It's not that big a deal. You're making something out of nothing. I was in total control."

Then, he switched gears and said, "You don't understand. My friends don't understand. Nobody gets it. I don't drink and smoke weed for the same reasons other guys do. I'm not trying to get wasted. I have totally different reasons."

Wanting to understand I asked, "Michael, do you get wasted to avoid the craziness at home?"

He'd seen some scary stuff and avoided talking about it. It seemed reasonable that substance abuse was his method of escape.

"That might be part of it, but only a small part. There are other things, other reasons, but I don't want to talk about them. I'll work it out. That's what I am doing. I'm working it out."

Mark said to him, "You need to tell us what's going on, Michael. We're your parents and we want to help you make the right choices."

"They're my choices to make, and no matter how many questions you ask I'm not going to talk about it, at least not now." He stood firm.

So we laid down the law. Absolutely no drugs or alcohol. He could no longer spend the night at other people's houses and his grades had to come up. When he came home at midnight (a curfew he'd not yet missed), he'd take a breathalyzer test. We also warned him that we would test his urine for marijuana beginning in a month, by which time prior use would no longer show up in his system. He complained, but not as fiercely as I'd expected. I ordered drug and alcohol testing supplies off the Internet.

Before the testing supplies made it through the mail to our house, we got a phone call from the local sheriff telling us Michael had been arrested along with several other teens. He asked us to come pick him up. Mark and I drove down the highway and entered the sheriff substation, feeling a mixture of anger and concern. Michael was not high or drunk. In fact, he was quiet and respectful. He was charged with "minor in possession of tobacco" and "possession of drug paraphernalia."

The officer explained what had happened. He saw a car filled with teens, following it as a matter of policy. One of the taillights was out and then someone threw a cigarette out the window. Since the occupants appeared to be under eighteen, the sheriff had reason to pull them over. He ordered them out of the car and told them to empty their pockets. Michael had a pack of cigarettes, a lighter, and a marijuana pipe. That was enough to make an arrest.

We signed him out, took him home, and blew up. Both Mark and I were amazed at his stupidity and bold disregard for our recently reinforced rules. He insisted that he hadn't smoked pot, but that point seemed moot. He had the pipe in his pocket.

Within a couple of weeks Michael and I were required to attend a hearing for the charges, which were dropped once he completed a tobacco diversion program and community service. He was a little miffed that Mark and I hadn't hired a lawyer and gotten him off, as some of the other parents had. I was more than a little miffed that my son had made choices that resulted in my having to spend time in unsavory places I'd never imagined I would visit. I was angry and uncomfortable picking him up from the sheriff's office, going to juvenile court, taking him to the county-funded lab for urine drops. I did not want to assume any more responsibility for his choices, and neither did Mark. He needed to bear the consequences of his actions.

Michael fulfilled the requirements of the diversion program, and we put the incident behind us. We clamped down harder than ever, but soon discovered that the tough approach was not going to work. I regularly searched his things and continued to find eye drops, used baggies, lighters, rolling papers, and other telling items. Ultimately, he stopped try to hide them, leaving paraphernalia on his nightstand in complete defiance of our agreement.

We stopped letting him go out, then discovered that he left the house after we were asleep. We clamped down harder. He magnified his deceptions. One night we caught him sneaking back into the house. He announced that he wasn't going to stop smoking weed no matter what we did. He tried to explain that he smoked just to feel "normal" and that he didn't want to stop. Now convinced that Bipolar Disorder was the culprit behind the past few months' turmoil, I broached the subject. This infuriated him.

"I am nothing like Chloe. I am not crazy. That has nothing to do with it. Just leave me alone."

29
May 2002

"But I am constitutionally sensitive — nervous in a very unusual degree. I became insane, with long periods of horrible insanity. During these fits of absolute unconsciousness, I drank, God knows how much or how long. As a matter of course, my enemies referred the insanity to the drink rather the drink to the insanity."
— Edgar Allan Poe

As the weeks passed, Michael continued to use and we knew it. Then other disturbing signs emerged. Gregarious from birth, he spent an inordinate amount of time alone. On several occasions, I discovered him sobbing into his pillow. Then the sadness deepened and I found him lying on his back staring at the ceiling, tears silently running down his face and into his ears. I made an appointment with the doctor, and surprisingly, he was willing to go.

Michael was deeply depressed. I empathized and wanted him to experience the miraculous relief I felt after taking Zoloft. I knew an antidepressant would either make him feel better or induce mania, but it was clear that he needed medication in order to recover. Our primary care physician, however, took a hard line approach. Despite our family history, Dr. Sander refused to treat him for depression because of his ongoing substance abuse. She insisted that he enter a treatment center or rehab program. I agreed with her, but thought the depression required concurrent treatment. Despite my pleas, she declined to authorize treatment until he began a program.

When Mark got home from work that night, we talked about the doctor's advice. He thought she overreacted and suggested we get a new family doctor. Then I said something that shocked even me.

"Mark, Michael needs help. This is not normal teenage behavior. This is not my problem. It is not the doctor's problem. Michael is in trouble. He needs help and he won't cooperate if he thinks you don't see a problem. If you can't support me and help get him some help, I'm leaving. I love you both too much to stay and watch my son destroy himself. It's too painful. I won't do it any more."

Even as the words left my mouth, I couldn't believe what I was saying, and Mark couldn't believe his ears.

"I'll do whatever you want me to do. I'll do whatever you need, Katie. Let's figure this out together. Just don't leave me."

I called our insurance carrier who suggested several intensive outpatient programs in our area, and took Michael for an initial evaluation at a local facility in early May of 2002. He and I were interviewed separately and then together.

If Michael was accepted into the program, Mark would be interviewed before we began. During my session, I shared my gut feeling that Michael had Bipolar Disorder. When we met together for the final combined interview, the intake counselor brought up that possibility to Michael. Unlike previous conversations on the subject, he didn't patently reject her suggestion, but said he thought he was just depressed.

The counselor asked us several more questions then candidly said, "Michael, I'm not convinced you're ready to work on your substance abuse issues. I don't think you've admitted to yourself that you have a problem with drugs and alcohol, although you admit that you feel pretty bad and want to feel better. Knowing that, and knowing your family history of mental illness, I'm apprehensive about admitting you. I think you need an inpatient placement, but I'm willing to give it a try if you're willing to commit."

"I can't believe you think I need to be put away," Michael responded. "I want to feel better. I'm tired of feeling like crap all the time. If I have to do this to feel better, then I'll do it."

Michael and I were both surprised that she believed an inpatient program was more appropriate. I thought it was rather extreme and felt certain we could find both the underlying cause and solution in an outpatient program. During the drive home, we talked about it and Michael seemed motivated to feel better.

I knew he'd succeed. As soon as he finished the school year and Mark went through his portion of the intake interview process, we commenced our six-month, thrice-weekly rehab stint.

During the months that we participated in the rehab program with Michael, Chloe focused on recovery, too. She had cycled so rapidly for so long that her brain was a wreck. Dr. Kahil insisted that she remain free of other responsibilities, including school or work, in order to heal from the preceding months' manic episode. She stayed home most of the time, occasionally meeting friends for an evening out. Thankfully, she remained stable enough to avoid another hospitalization.

Monica went to school, played basketball, soccer, and volleyball, participated in drama, and hung out with her friends now and then. Mark and I made sure we were at her sporting and school events, often dividing up so that one of us was at family group for Michael's rehab program, too.

We were spread thin and distracted, and because Monica wasn't in crisis, she wasn't our primary focus. I was, and always will be, thankful that she came to this life independent and self-sufficient. Even though she was very young, she understood the demands of Chloe's and Michael's situations and accepted that her dad and I were doing the best we could. She never complained and often told us we didn't need to worry about making it to her activities.

Despite those comments, Mark and I were determined to be there for her. Not only did we want to make sure Monica didn't get lost in the chaos, we also loved the normalcy of spending time with her and enjoying her company. Many times I thanked God that we had her to help balance our life's experiences. My love for each of my three children is vast and immeasurable, but if I hadn't had a child without serious mental illness, I'd have had difficulty understanding my life's purpose, the reasons for it all. I'm not sure I could have grown through the challenges. Monica's birth, her existence in our family was, *is*, a gift.

30

Early Summer 2002

"This world is a school, designed to make us strong and help us learn to make wise choices. We continually are tested. What is the prize? A surprising one, as it may not look like much in the world, but there is nothing greater: awareness of ourselves as a Soul having experiences in this world, learning, growing, and ultimately, returning to our home in Spirit."

—John-Roger

In an effort to reinforce my spiritual and emotional self, I began practicing meditation and relaxation. For at least thirty minutes each day, I sat quietly cross-legged, focusing within. I released my mind from the process of thought and tried to access the stillness that lay inside of me. Often, thoughts and ideas would move through my mind, and I learned to observe them without judgment or concern, without joining them in an internal conversation. I liken the process to the silent, solitary act of watching clouds drift across a bright blue sky. This practice rejuvenated me.

This routine relieved the physical symptoms of stress, helped me assess my values, release anger and judgment, and live with greater awareness. It also drew me closer to God and helped me to access my spirituality at an ever-deepening level. Quite simply, meditation improved me.

As I improved, I became more appreciative of others, more aware of their goodness. As I valued myself more, I also valued others more. I began to see the world through clearer, more accepting eyes. It's ironic that my children's illnesses created the avenue by which I learned to feel at ease with individual uniqueness. I released unfulfilled expectations and acknowledged my children's rights to make choices, even if mine might be different. I again embraced the strange truth that, without challenges, none of us would develop our strength and character.

Because we perpetually talked about Chloe's and Michael's treatments, comparing our perceptions of each situation, and because the illness that triggered those treatments nearly tore us apart, Mark and I learned to communicate better than ever before. We made concerted efforts to talk openly and honestly, until we each felt understood by the other. Sometimes this was unreasonably hard. We carefully chose our words in order to communicate our feelings without demeaning the other. Often one of us bit our tongue and suppressed automatic reactions while the other muddled through the difficult process of articulating confusing and sensitive ideas.

We reverted to our college psychology training, using "I" statements to explain how we felt, avoiding easy-to-use and accusatory "you" statements. It was work. It would have been easy to walk away and leave the other partner holding the bag. Nevertheless, neither of us walked, and because we stayed and put forth the effort, we are greatly blessed, our relationship incredibly enriched.

Mark and I have always had an unusually close and supportive partnership, yet the challenges of chronic illness and substance abuse nearly pushed us to the breaking point. We felt the powerful pressure that families like ours withstand, and understand the sad statistics on separation and divorce. I'm grateful the strength of our love and commitment outweighed other possibilities. We weathered the harshest storms and know that we can keep ourselves, and then one another, afloat. Still, we often felt frustrated, challenged, and stretched to our limits.

Even bigger obstacles loomed ahead.

31
Summer 2002

"Ah, yes, the sea is still and deep
All things within its bosom sleep.
A single step, and all is o'er,
A plunge, a bubble, and no more."
— Henry Wadsworth Longfellow

By the middle of July 2002, the children were settling in. Two months had passed since Chloe's hospitalization and we'd been in Michael's rehab program for nearly as long. He seemed to be making a serious effort and the counselors were pleased with his progress. From the other families in the group, Mark and I learned a lot about enabling behaviors, medical perspectives, and the similarities our children shared. Although the program was time-consuming, the commitment rewarded us with knowledge and skills we'd have developed no other way.

I continued to push for medication management of the depression, which was worsening, but the director of the treatment facility and our family doctor agreed that Michael had to be substance-free before taking any medication. This meant several more weeks for residual elements to leave his body. Time and again, I was told to be patient.

The girls could have joined us in the family sessions, but I wondered if Chloe was stable enough to handle the emotional intensity and deal appropriately with some of the topics. Michael didn't want his sisters to hear the details of some of his activities and thought he might hold back if they were there. I left it up to them. I was glad when they declined participation, choosing to hang out together when we three left for several hours every Monday, Wednesday, and Saturday. It would be harder to deal with five sets of issues. Three was tough enough.

From my journal on July 3, 2002: "God grant me the serenity to accept the things I cannot change, the courage to change the things I can, and the wisdom to know the difference."

At four o'clock one July morning, I awoke with a start, drenched in sweat and thirsty. While I was in the kitchen getting a glass of water, the phone rang and Mark picked it up. It was the sheriff.

Michael, whom we thought was staying with a friend for the first time since we cracked down on him, had been in an accident and arrested. He was charged with, among other things, DUI. We dressed and made the five-minute drive to the station, passing the crashed car along the way. The arresting officer met us at the front door.

"You should know that your son is extremely intoxicated and threatening suicide. Usually we take them straight to the hospital when they're like this, but since he's a minor and you both agreed to pick him up, I'm releasing him to your custody."

When Michael emerged from the holding area, he erupted into uncontrollable sobs. In a voice that was heavy with liquor and difficult to understand, he wept, "I'm so sorry guys. I really messed up. I ruined my car. I'm such a screw-up. I can't do anything right. I'm so sorry. I don't know why you guys put up with me."

Mark asked, "Michael, what happened? We saw the car. How did you crash it? Why were you driving at this time of night? You were supposed to be at Nathan's."

"I know. I know. I was anxious and couldn't sleep. I thought if I got home and in my own bed, I'd be okay. When I came up the highway, a coyote or something ran in front of me and I swerved to miss it. I hit the shoulder and lost it. The car just spun out of control."

Even though his speech was ridiculously slurred, and he was so wasted he drooled as he talked, Michael's story made sense. The way he described the accident was verified by what we had seen when we passed the car wedged between two trees on the shoulder of the highway. I immediately felt some compassion, knowing fear and anxiety had placed him behind the wheel of the car. Equally concerning was what had driven him to, again, get so trashed. Looking back now, I wonder why we allowed Michael to have access to a car. Oddly, I can't explain why. In hindsight, we were foolish.

As we finished with the sheriff and walked out the door, Michael put his arms around both Mark and me and said: "I love you guys and the girls very much. What I've done, and what I'm going to do, isn't a reflection on you. It's all me. It's all inside of me. It's just me."

We took him home and for the next two hours he cried, cursed, and pounded his fists against his bedroom wall and his own head. He tried to convince us to go back to bed, and when that did not work, he tried to provoke Mark to hit him. Then he got Chloe's keys and headed for the door, but he was still wasted and physically out of control, making it easy for me to hold him back. When I stopped him, he shouted, "Fine, I'll kill myself in front of you. Is that what you want?"

My thoughts raced. "No. This is not what I want. I want my children to be healthy. I want never to deal with the fear that one of them might take his or her own life. I want them free of the demons that dwell within their brains, free of misfiring electrical impulses, chemical shortages, or miscommunicated signals. Whatever it is, I want it gone."

I knew it would not simply go away, so I told Michael how much we loved him. We assured him that nothing was so bad we could not overcome it, that he could never do anything that would cost him our love. We poured out our hearts hoping to reach him, hoping to pull him back from the edge, hoping to save him from himself.

By 6:45 a.m., he fell into an exhausted sleep and didn't awaken for hours. However, before he was able to relax to that point, he told us that he'd considered suicide many times, dating back to grade school. "Life is no good. It's not worth living," he said.

It broke my heart to see him in such turmoil. I loved him so much and again found myself questioning why my children endured such suffering. It was clear that the drugs and alcohol were efforts at self-medication, and now I understood his meaning when he said the reasons he "used" were far different from his friends'. Many times, he had said he got high or drunk just to feel "okay." The truth was clear.

When Michael woke up, he was still talking about suicide, so I told Chloe to lock up all of her medications. Unfortunately, he was one step ahead of us and had already taken what remained of a Lorazapam prescription she no longer used. This act, in itself, illustrated Michael's strength of character and kind heart. He sifted through all of the prescription bottles and selected the one that Chloe no longer needed, so its absence would neither affect her medical routine nor endanger her health. Even when entangled in a quagmire of depression and hopelessness, he considered her needs.

Checking on Michael every ten to fifteen minutes, I noticed his eyes looked different and his speech was slightly slurred. I told Chloe to recheck her meds and she discovered the empty bottle. She figured he'd taken about seventy-five one-mg. tablets. We dashed to the emergency room where Michael was immediately admitted, put on an IV drip, and given medication to counteract the respiratory distress the overdose caused.

Angry that we had interfered, Michael grew verbally and physically combative, threatening, foul-mouthed, and angry. I recognized suicidal anxiety and mania much like Chloe had suffered a year before. The similarities in the manifestation of their illnesses, despite the differences in their personalities and choices, amazed me.

Once Michael's vitals were stabilized, the attending physician moved him from the pediatric emergency area to the cardiac intensive care wing so the staff could monitor his respiration and heartbeat. While there, he displayed odd behaviors that I'd never witnessed before. Several of his friends came to see him and the nursing staff allowed them in his room. His persona transformed before our eyes.

To the girls, he was flirtatious and charming, "Get up on this bed with me and rub my back. That's what I'm talking about." And to another, "You know you want to rub my feet. That's right. You're perfect. That's good. Yeah." He smiled, touched their hands and faces, and nuzzled their necks. I felt embarrassed by the intimacy. Then he changed again, for the worse. Michael began to act bold and macho.

"I'm the man. I AM the man and I'm not gonna stay here. I'm goin' out with a bang. Ain't nobody gonna mess with me.

I'm not gonna do this. I'm outta here, man, I'm gone. I'm gonna get outta this bed and run. I'm on the run."

He grew cocky as his voice grew louder, and became physically agitated, opening and closing his fists, tightening his jaw, and speaking through clenched teeth. His eyes went wild, wide open, and glassy. He took on the mannerisms and dialect of action movie bad guys, using profoundly foul language. To the boys, "You guys gotta fuckin' help me out here. I gotta get out. These motha-fuckas can't keep me here. Let's go. We'll take 'em on. We'll fuckin' mess 'em up, bro." His volume and tone served as alarms and the doctor quickly entered the room.

"Michael, this is unacceptable. If you do not stop, your friends will have to leave and I'll bring in security."

"Bring it on, bitch. Bring it on, cuz I'm outta here." Then he jumped out of the bed, throwing himself at the window.

The minute Michael leapt out of the bed, Mark leapt, too. He and two of the boys managed to keep Michael from going through the glass. He collapsed into tears, but continued to thrash his arms, trying to free himself from their grip. "God damn it. Let me die. Why won't you just let me die? I'm not worth it. I'm no good. Let me die."

We were stunned. As Mark jumped to subdue Michael, the doctor called security. Two guards entered the room and helped Mark get Michael back on the bed. We sent his friends out, and most of them went home.

"Get off that bed again, Michael, and I'll have you restrained," the doctor told him, "and that's not something you want. I'll have security tie you to that bed."

"I'm cool, man. I'm cool. I'm sorry. That was my bad, man, my bad. I won't do it again."

We all knew he was lying.

For the next few minutes, Michael lay on the bed, looking from face to face, assessing the situation. He didn't talk to anybody and nobody talked to him. We were in shock. When the room felt a little less electric, less charged, Michael spoke, "I'm sorry. That was out of line. I'll be okay now. It'll be okay."

At the same time, however, he repeatedly glanced back and forth between the security guards and the window. I knew he was going to try it again. As I opened my mouth to utter a warning, he jumped. The security guards saw it coming, too, and were right on top of him. They pinned Michael down, called for assistance, and led him to the bed. Michael fought back, swinging his fists and fighting for his life. Before it was over, it took the doctor, a nurse, and four security officers to subdue him.

He was placed in full restraints, and injected with a "chemical straitjacket" containing Haldol. I couldn't hold back my tears as the surrealistic scene played out. I felt detached from the situation, yet enmeshed in the drama. I prayed that he'd sleep deeply and through the night so he wouldn't feel frightened and alone. He'd grown afraid to sleep alone lately, sure that he was in danger. This was the paranoia that drove him to leave his friend's house the night before, and drive drunk. I yearned for him to experience some relief.

From my journal: "Seeing Michael so brutally treated broke my heart into a million little pieces that scattered through my chest and paralyzed my lungs. I forced myself to breathe. I could do nothing but send powerful prayers of love and comfort, hoping my energy would seep through the walls to embrace, inform, and protect him. I know that I can't protect him, and I don't like that very much. Please, God, let him feel my love."

The next day Mark and I visited Michael in the psychiatric hospital where he was under suicide watch. He remained angry and defiant, wanting to know why we put him there. He was still irrational, vacillating between verbal aggressions and crying like a toddler. When he cried, I cried, and at the sight of my tears, he cried harder, pleading, "Don't cry, Mama, don't waste your tears on me."

His pain was palpable. We couldn't do anything. I yearned for his liberation from inner turmoil. We stayed the allotted hour. Each night we returned for a brief visit. Each night we felt increasingly encouraged as Michael emerged from behind the persona that masked his true self. At every visit he seemed a little less frantic, a little less agitated, a little more like his old self.

After six days in the psychiatric hospital, Michael left with prescriptions for Effexor XR and Trazadone, diagnosed, like Chloe, with Bipolar Disorder. Faced with the reality that Michael, too, was seriously mentally ill, Mark despaired. For reasons he's never been able to articulate, he found it more difficult to accept Michael's illness than it had been to accept Chloe's. Was it because he was a boy, or was it simply the weight of yet another child fallen ill? I don't know. He never said.

Whatever the reason, Mark was withdrawn and deeply saddened for quite some time. It took weeks for him to come out of the funk. (A few years later, when my dear friend Tina died, I experienced the same sensations and made the connection that Mark was literally going through the grieving process.) During that time, I questioned many things, not the least of which was, quite simply, how would this all turn out?

I also wondered at our bad luck. Why had not one, but two, of our children been cursed with Bipolar Disorder? When I read statistics suggesting that Monica had a seventy-five percent chance of developing the disorder, I felt infuriated, inadequate, and exhausted. I grieved all over again, as I had with Chloe's diagnosis. Mark and I were adrift in the middle of an ocean with no lifebuoys, while our children slipped below the water line, bobbing up and then under, over and over again. How many times could they resurface? Where would they find the strength? I doubted our ability to navigate the treacherous waters and keep them afloat. I feared the outcome if things did not get better.

Both girls were elated when Michael returned home. Chloe understood the isolation and fear that accompanied hospitalization, and Monica idolized and missed him. Michael began seeing a psychiatrist once a week for medication management, and we returned to the outpatient program. At least now the situation was defined—my two oldest children were each diagnosed with Juvenile Onset Bipolar Disorder at age seventeen. Monica expressed great fear about turning seventeen. I appreciated and shared her fear.

Like a gift from God, family friends called the next day and invited Monica for a week in Newport Beach. It was perfect. We'd cancelled our annual trip to the beach in order to complete the rehab program and provide stability for Chloe. This invitation offered exactly what Monica needed. I was grateful for the generosity of that family, for their willingness to listen to their hearts and open their arms.

32
August 2002

"Do not attempt to hide things which cannot be hid."
— Aesop

Michael responded to his medications more quickly than Chloe ever had. The mixed state of agitation and deep depression subsided and, just days after reaching therapeutic doses, he felt like himself. Although paranoia and anxiety still plagued him, the anger and aggression existed only in painful memories of the recent past. Now that we had two children with the same diagnosis, we saw, despite common symptoms, how differently Bipolar Disorder presents itself in each individual it strikes.

The week that Monica was gone, Michael took the assessments necessary for admittance to the local junior college. He was a high school senior, but Michael, Mark, the high school principal, and I agreed that returning to campus in the fall would not be in his best interest. He would go to the JC for a semester as a dually enrolled student and then reassess in December.

At the same time, we filled out reams of forms and collected documentation to maintain Chloe as a dependent on Mark's insurance plan because of the disabling nature of her illness. The university had contacted the Social Security Administration on her behalf and we were plowing through the paperwork they required. During one of a dozen trips across town to collect information and signatures, I thought about Monica playing on a beach and felt thankful that she was enjoying a respite from the chaos that had become our lives.

Just two weeks later, in August of 2002, our extended family expected us in Northern California for a wedding. After deliberating for days, Mark and I decided to stick to the plan, mostly because it included several days in San Francisco, which we knew the children would love. The challenging element was, in the end, not as difficult as we thought it would be. We had not yet told most of the extended family about Chloe's and Michael's illness.

Chloe was stable and somewhat in control of her moods, but she continued to struggle with severe anxiety and sleeplessness, made physically apparent by chain-smoking and a negative attitude. Michael was vastly improved but, like Chloe, still felt terribly anxious much of the time and continued to be hounded by relentless paranoia. Suspicious of people and things, he often felt threatened or unsafe. Despite their improvement, it was apparent that something was wrong.

Fearing we'd be forced to spill the beans, Mark and I talked about what to do and decided to be honest. Through no fault of their own, our children had Bipolar Disorder, and we decided it was important for everybody's recovery and their long-term stability that we stop hiding behind a veil of guilt or shame. We owed our children that much. When the inevitable questions arose we told the truth and our family, while sheepish and uncertain, was kind and supportive. We learned that sometimes we create problems for ourselves where none exists.

After spending time with family, we drove to San Francisco. We stayed in a posh hotel and ate great food. We immersed ourselves in that marvelous city, riding trolley cars and busses, and taking in the sights. We spent an afternoon at Alcatraz, wandered through gardens and museums, shopped in unusual stores, and walked for miles and miles. It felt good to breathe the sea air and hang out together as a family. There was only one glitch in the trip.

As we walked and talked in our little group of five, Michael's paranoia and anxiety grew painfully obvious. He thought people, especially homeless men, were talking about him, or staring at him, or challenging him to fight. By each day's end, he was wild-eyed and fidgety, smoking more than normal, unable to stand or sit still, and constantly looking over his shoulder.

A couple of times Mark had to lead him away from escalating verbal exchanges with men on the street. We saw how easily discord and violence could rule the lives of the mentally ill, and knew we must continue to help Chloe and Michael improve their health and make wise choices. We also developed compassion for the millions of homeless people living on the streets, realizing that many were at the mercy of their own minds just as sure as they were at the mercy of the elements. Even though those moments frightened us, we had a wonderful time together and grew closer after being torn apart.

One factor adding to the trip's pleasure was Chloe's significant improvement. We could attribute it to one thing. Several weeks earlier, I had injured my back while trimming trees. X-rays revealed arthritis in my neck and spine, and the doctor prescribed physical therapy three times a week. Following that regimen, I felt slow, minimal improvement.

A friend recommended I try craniosacral therapy, a hands-on, subtle energy healing treatment, much less intense than chiropractic work, which allows the body to release stored tension and heal itself. I made an appointment with a local practitioner and felt such improvement after one session that I continued with weekly appointments, eliminating the physical therapy.

I wondered how craniosacral therapy would affect Chloe and her illness, so I encouraged her to try it. After a few treatments, she knew greater stability than she had in some time, slept better, and needed fewer therapy sessions with Maria. We actually relate the beginning of her long-term increased wellness to this rarely used healing method. She was finally feeling relief from her most nagging symptoms, and that relief translated into a positive change in our family dynamics.

I also think that our changing attitudes, healing intentions, and attempts to let go of judgment profoundly affected us. I continued with daily prayerful meditation, as well as research and study about Bipolar Disorder and its satellite issues. Mark, Michael, and I kept up with the parent and family sessions in the treatment program. We stopped blaming, learned greater acceptance, and recognized blessings. Old habits and patterns still emerged, but we each changed for the better.

During the last two weeks of August 2002, Monica began high school, Michael started at the community college, and

Chloe continued to improve. We even talked about the possibility of her returning to the university in a few months. She still had days when she couldn't get out of bed, but they were rare. More often, she battled anxiety and low-level mania, but was learning how to live with their presence. She took good care of Molly, taking her to the park and for walks. She helped drive Monica to and from volleyball and soccer practice, and was more willing to do things around the house. Most significantly, her tension and anxiety abated and she argued less often.

We breezed through three or four weeks like this, and then, as is so frustratingly typical of destabilized Bipolar Disorder, she began a rapid downward spiral. I stopped journaling again and my calendar pages contain lists like:

CALL:
- Mental health insurance
- In Balance (another outpatient program)
- Michael's psychiatrist
- Dr. Kahil
- Dr. David (new psychiatrist)
- Maria
- Chuck (Michael's new therapist)

Chloe was still doing craniosacral therapy every week, and returned to weekly appointments with Maria, too. The occurrence of Dr. David's name on my lists indicates when Chloe grew tired of not getting better and taking more and more medications. She decided that Dr. Kahil had been great for a while, but since his practice centered on children, perhaps he no longer offered what she needed. She sought out a new psychiatrist. Michael also refused to see his doctor again, so I searched for someone who might take them both. Dr. David was willing to do that. Of course, we were still going to intensive outpatient therapy three times a week.

As soon as Chloe began with Dr. David, she felt encouraged. Dr. David thought she was on too many meds and took her off some immediately, while weaning her off others. She wanted to try new prescriptions when her system was clear of the old. She assured Chloe that she had treated more challenging cases and that, in time, Chloe could be stable and independent. Chloe and I both left her office feeling better about her prognosis than perhaps we ever had.

Michael's situation was progressing, too. He finally went to court for the DUI he received in July and was placed on probation. He was assigned a probation officer and ordered to go to "Drunk Driving School," meet with *Mothers Against Drunk Drivers*, perform community service, and spend twenty-four hours in jail. He was also required to continue drug and alcohol treatment, go for drug testing two to three times a week, and pay damages for the sign he hit when he crashed his car. He couldn't drive until he turned eighteen in March, which meant that I'd continue to drive him to school, doctor's appointments, and other commitments for six more months. We made another trip to the emergency room when he nearly severed a finger while running a power saw at a part-time job. It is not surprising I stopped writing in my journal.

Then Michael refused to continue in the intensive outpatient drug and alcohol treatment program. I was somewhat relieved since it was a major commitment, and after a period during which we'd all benefited, Michael didn't seem to be improving. He'd been in the program so long he knew how to work it. That old Michael charm was hard at work. He knew what to say, he knew how to act. He needed a program that addressed both mental illness and substance abuse. This wasn't it.

We needed a different approach and since he was court-ordered to receive some form of treatment, he agreed to see a highly touted therapist. When we met with the director of the treatment facility for an exit interview, he candidly admitted that his program had not helped Michael and recommended inpatient treatment to us as well as our insurance case manager. He thought Michael was on a suicide mission that required serious intervention. Our family doctor made the same suggestion.

Despite the professional opinions that Michael be hospitalized, neither Mark nor I was ready to take that step. Our (perhaps misguided) love and commitment to him still overshadowed his need for round-the-clock care. We held out hope that living at home and regular appointments with both a psychiatrist and a therapist would adequately address his needs. It was a pipe dream, but we needed more time to come to terms with what had to be done.

Several weeks later Dr. David called me at home just after we returned from his regular appointment with her. She wanted to speak on the phone rather than in Michael's presence after his appointment.

"Michael bullied me into giving him another prescription for the anti-anxiety medication he's been taking. I didn't want to prescribe any more because he's gone through it too quickly, but I have to tell you, I felt threatened. I gave in and wrote a prescription, but it's the last time. It was clearly drug-seeking behavior. If he comes at me with that kind of aggression again, I won't continue to treat him. This incident makes it clear to me that he needs inpatient treatment for substance abuse as well as Bipolar Disorder, and that's what I'll recommend when I speak with his insurance case worker later today."

I couldn't believe what she was saying. Although I didn't articulate my thoughts, I questioned her honesty and integrity. Somehow I'd temporarily forgotten how aggressive he'd been after the last failed suicide attempt. The picture she painted was not the Michael I wanted to know. My Michael wasn't a bully. He was concerned about other people's feelings and well-being. Since he was little he'd stood up for underdogs, the children whom bullies victimized.

I was certain she'd misunderstood, or misread, or missed something. She noticed my trepidation and made it clear that Michael was seriously ill. She wanted him under constant observation so that his illness, medication side effects, and addiction-related behaviors could be separated and understood. The seriousness of his situation escalated again.

Despite the challenges regarding Michael's health and behavior, his grades had improved and he wanted to spend his last semester on the high school campus so he could participate in graduation ceremonies. Mark and I hesitated to make that move, but scheduled an appointment with his principal to discuss options. She, too, was unconvinced that Michael was well enough to return to the pressures of a high

school campus, but she wanted to offer him every
opportunity to succeed, and was willing to try. We re-
enrolled him, met with his counselor to register for classes,
and looked forward with trepidation. Very soon, our
uneasiness met disaster head-on.

33
Late 2002

"You know what charm is:
A way of getting the answer yes without having asked any clear
question."
— Albert Camus

Predictably, I stopped making daily journal entries when our lives became too demanding, too sad. Venturing back through my memories of late 2002, visions of tears and fears overwhelm me. Chloe was improving, but Dr. David had not yet discovered the best blend of medications to manage her mental health. The low-level mania she experienced most days caused irritability, grandiosity, assertiveness, and tactlessness. To her credit, she worked closely with Maria to recognize her symptoms and learn to hold them at bay, but she was just developing this self-analysis and had not incorporated it into her daily interactions as well as she ultimately would.

Chloe became Michael's greatest critic, and the mounting fear she felt around him drove her racing thoughts. She was angry that he used drugs and alcohol since she struggled with similar challenges without considering those options. She was disappointed in the way he handled his challenges and disappointed in the way Mark and I handled him. As much as she feared for her own safety, she hated the way Michael treated me, and was afraid that he might hurt me.

Most of our conversations were about Michael and her fears about what he might do to himself, or to her, or to me.

"Mom, I can't believe the way he treats you, and I can't believe Dad lets him get away with it. You never would have let me act that way. He's out of control. You have to put him in the hospital."

Other times, "I don't trust him not to hurt you, Mom, or not to hurt me. I don't feel safe here any more. I'm not sure he won't do something stupid or dangerous."

Consequences be damned, Michael continued making unhealthy choices. I never knew if he was high, drunk, or mentally off-balance. Futilely, I dissected his every word and action trying to get a handle on what was going on. I read some of his writing from that period, catching a brief glimpse into his inner world. It was sad. It was frightening.

"I'm gonna go out with a bang. I will try anything, do everything, experience every crazy thing I have ever thought of doing. And then I'll be done. I'll just die."

His poetry was reminiscent of gangster rap laced with foul language and carefully crafted rhymes. It roared off the pages creating images of disappointment and fear. In writings, he insisted that he could not be the person everybody wanted him to be. He felt like a constant disappointment to others, as if his essential self was not in line with the world's standards. After watching Chloe struggle through years of unsuccessful attempts to manage her mental illness, he wanted none of the medical approach. He took some of his meds, but not others. He took other substances to alleviate anxiety or insomnia, or provide a temporary escape.

Several parents called me to voice concerns over the substance abuse Michael and their sons seemed to be involved in. His closest friends continued to be concerned about him, too. I received telephone calls from no less than a half-dozen of them as they shared their observations and worries, and offered an abundance of love and support to Michael and to us. I learned that some of the kids I considered the worst influences over Michael were actually among those who tried valiantly to help him. I also learned that Michael, my son, my love, my pride and joy, was the kid others should avoid.

"I'm the bad one, Mom. I'm the one who has power over everyone else."

Power was one way to describe what Michael had. Charisma...Charm...Magnetism...They all applied. I recall, "Michael's charm will be his downfall." A very sensitive friend explained, "He will do great good in this world, or he will do great evil. Whatever Michael chooses to do, it will be big. But only he can choose how he will use his power." These comments, despite being esoteric, made sense to me. I shared them with Michael in an attempt to appeal to the goodness that I knew dwelled in his core. I spoke to the sweet boy I had always known.

"That's the person you want me to be," he told me. "That's not the person I am. I do not want to live the dull existence you have in mind. I want more."

Throughout this time, Michael still showed us loving kindness. Unlike many young people struggling with similar circumstances, he told us he loved us and sought hugs and closeness. Despite recent transformations and occurrences of anger and hostility, he still interacted in warm and delightful ways.

He was the true embodiment of Dr. Jekyll and Mr. Hyde. I felt at a loss, and that was probably the best feeling I could have had, because it enabled me to accept Michael's right to make his own choices and realize my powerlessness. He had been right all along. He was the one with the power, but as his mother, I wanted to continue in a parental role that he'd outgrown. Waves of sadness washed over me, but when the tide turned, I realized peace as I finally accepted what was. As he grew more and more unbalanced and ill, Mark and I battened down the hatches for the emotional storm that now seemed inevitable.

Since I avoided writing during this painful time, I made this entry in my journal several months after the fact: "In November and December Michael's moods, attitudes, and behaviors deteriorated. He challenged everyone around him. He was verbally contrary and combative. He tried to engage family, friends, and acquaintances in debates, arguments, and physical altercations.

He was subtly and physically challenging toward Chloe and me. He clenched his fists, puffed up his chest, leaned in, and raised his voice. I began to feel insecure and unsafe around him. This saddened me deeply. I love this boy so much, and find it difficult to accept that he threatened me. Then he'd behave lovingly and kindly, and I'd doubt myself all over again."

In late November, 2002, Mark and I went to a dinner party just minutes from the house. Chloe and Monica were home and Michael's friends planned to pick him up to go play video games. Around nine o'clock one of the other boys called us, frantic. They were still at our house.

"Mrs. McLaughlin, you've gotta come home. Something's wrong with Michael. He's crazy. He keeps trying to get us to hit him. He's saying things that don't make sense. We don't know what to do."

We immediately went home.

When we arrived, Michael was moving stealthily around his friends, eyes wide open, jaw clenched, hands tightened into fists. He yelled, "Come on you pussies, hit me. You're so tough. Hit me. Let's see who's tough. Let's go." Mark pulled Michael away from the other boys, walking him outside.

I was angry. "What did he take? Were you drinking or doing drugs? Have you been smoking weed?"

"No. We swear. That's why this is so weird. We've seen Michael like this before and thought he was wasted. But we were here. We were playing video games and hanging out. None of us did anything or took anything, and he got like this. This is all Michael. That's why it's so freaking scary."

It took Mark and me several hours to settle Michael down, and the next day he was as baffled as we were by the behavior and its cause.

A few weeks later, on a mid-December Saturday evening, Mark and I dressed in formal attire and went to an annual charity ball, a highlight of the holiday season. We'd anticipated the special evening for weeks, buying formal wear, planning the day's preparations, and booking a room at the resort where the event was held. It felt like a mini-vacation and we were excited. Although still a bit edgy, Chloe was much improved, and Mark had a serious discussion with Michael about our expectations for the night. All three children gave assurances that they'd be fine, and we were only thirty minutes away.

We spent six delicious hours dancing, dining, and enjoying the good company and ourselves. When we got back to our room, red lights blinked on both cell phones and the room phone. All of them held variations of the same message: Michael was drinking. He and Chloe argued. He threatened her. She called the police. He left with friends. Nobody knew where he was. We threw our things into the car and left the hotel without checking out.

As we drove home, we spoke with both girls on the phone. Monica had called a friend whose mom came and picked her up. After Michael left, Chloe filed a report with the police and then went to her friend Eric's to spend the night. When we walked into the house, Michael was there and relatively calm. We three talked for quite a while. He was despondent, threatening suicide, and vowing to leave. Mark stayed up with him until he fell asleep at five o'clock the next morning. We were in over our heads.

From my journal: "How strange it is that we let this go on and on without taking greater action. We didn't want to 'put Michael away somewhere.' We love him so much, we were certain we could take better care of him. How? Why? What were we thinking? Who knows?"

Having spent the last year building a new house and selling the one we were in, we prepared to move just before Christmas. Although the construction process had been a welcome diversion from the craziness in our family, it was demanding and finally ending.

Maybe we thought we would get into the new house and our situation would magically change. We did a lot of magical thinking during those challenging times. We also tried to deal in practicalities and my calendar pages verify weekly telephone conversations with the insurance case manager, as well as names and phone numbers of inpatient facilities that treated dually diagnosed adolescents, where both the substance abuse and mental illness would be addressed.

Finding a program for Michael was more difficult than I'd anticipated. In addition to the complication of his age—he would be eighteen in just a few months—most facilities treated either substance abuse or mental illness, but had no functioning model for treating the whole person when the two coexisted. I still marvel at this ridiculous fact, since most mentally ill patients self-medicate and many develop addictions.

Dual diagnosis, the term applied to patients with both a mental illness and a history of substance abuse, has been on the books for decades. Based on a study done over twenty years ago, from 1980-1984, NAMI (The National Alliance on Mental Illness) estimates that sixty-one percent of individuals diagnosed with Bipolar Disorder also have substance abuse issues. Despite these overwhelming statistics and the fact that most clinicians verify co-morbid diagnoses (another term for dual diagnosis), few facilities have reliable processes or systems to deal with them. The medical approach to mental health so badly requires evolution and reform.

We moved on December 23, 2002. Within a week, the tension between Chloe and Michael grew beyond tolerability and she moved out, sharing a house with two friends who had an extra room. I was happy and supportive of the change because she and Michael had become one another's nemeses. Each of their symptomatic behaviors set off the other. Each directed their worst moods toward the other. As Michael's tone and voice grew more aggressive and angry, and his body language intentionally intimidated, Chloe no longer felt safe living under the same roof with him.

Sadly, I was not convinced that she was wrong. Wanting to guarantee everybody's well-being, I encouraged her to make the move. Happily, that move was also a hallmark and beginning point for Chloe's improved health and greater independence.

A week later, on January 7, 2003, we endured what would prove to be our greatest challenge to date.

34
January 2003

"I am groaning under the miseries of a diseased nervous System; a System of all others the most essential to our happiness – or the most productive of our Misery…"
— Robert Burns

Michael's anxiety and irritability catapulted. He became more tightly wound with each passing day. He stayed up later and later, fearful of being alone in his room, hearing noises outside, dreaming frightening dreams. Each morning he emerged with a drawn, pale face, dark circles, and red-rimmed eyes. Since he was off work for the holidays, Mark finally saw, day in and day out, what the rest of us had witnessed, and was dumbfounded by Michael's surliness.

Until now, Michael managed to control himself when his dad was around, perhaps in an effort to please and protect him. Later I learned that children and adolescents diagnosed with mental illnesses or disorders often keep up a false front with nearly everyone but their mothers or primary caretakers, as if they subconsciously know they'll be safe with that person no matter what they do. Michael seemed to have done this, but with Mark home all the time, the effort was too great, becoming impossible.

Michael argued with all of us, any of us, over the most trivial issues. He could tolerate no further change in his surroundings or routine, and grew angry if the details of his day were not as he anticipated. Opening the refrigerator and realizing the apple juice was gone threw him into a tizzy.

"Who drank all the apple juice?" he screamed one morning. "You guys know I drink apple juice when I get up in the morning. Why didn't you leave some for me? I can't believe it. I hate it here. You always do stuff like this to me. I swear, nobody has any respect for me. I always get screwed."

Eerily repeating Chloe's behavior of three years before, Michael could tolerate no noise, exploding at any loud sound. Since we had just moved into the new house, tradesmen were in and out completing the final touches. If this required a power tool or a lot of talking, Michael stormed out of the house and into the wilderness behind our property to escape what, to him, was cacophony.

If we changed plans or deviated from the routine, he became agitated. He would pace, smoke, and wonder aloud at our inability to stick to a plan. In short, he fell apart. Just as Chloe began cutting when her internal pain grew intolerable, Michael turned to self-mutilation. The knuckles on both hands bled from the wounds he inflicted on himself as he futilely pummeled walls and tree trunks. His forearms sported puss-oozing, red-yellow sores where he extinguished cigarettes in his own flesh. He was a walking, talking, open wound into which internal salt was continually being rubbed.

Mark and I agreed. Michael was in tremendous inner pain. Aside from getting him to therapy and medical appointments, we didn't know what to do. We'd talked about long-term hospitalization several times, and the notion so terrified Michael that we were unable to make that move. I finally leveled with Mark.

"I'm growing afraid of him. I never thought I'd say this, but I think he might hurt me. Sometimes he looks at me and it feels like he's somebody else. His eyes flash anger, almost hatred. He's another person, and I'm not sure I'm safe when that person emerges."

Mark acknowledged that he'd seen it, too, and we agreed that I would have no choice but to call the sheriff if I ever felt at risk. I hoped I wouldn't have to do that. It seemed like such a betrayal of parental love. We wanted him to get better, and struggled with the fact that such a simple desire seemed so impossible to achieve.

Then, on a January day, things got worse rather than better. Michael quietly went through the morning and afternoon and invited his girlfriend over in the evening. Mark and I were in the family room directly adjacent to his bedroom, where he and Tiffany watched a movie and played an X-Box game. For a couple of hours we heard their muffled voices and thought they were having a good time until Michael suddenly began to yell, "Fuck you, bitch. Get the fuck out of my house. You little whore. Go on. Get the fuck out."

Tiffany charged through his bedroom door with Michael right behind her. Mark and I leapt up from the sofa just as Michael grabbed Tiffany's arm. He roughly led her through the family room, opened the door, and pushed her out.

"You fucking bitch. You cheated on me," he shouted after her. "You're nothing but a whore. I knew you'd cheat on me. I should have listened when everybody said you were nothing but a dirty slut."

Then he slammed the door and retreated to his room, Tiffany gazing at us through the glass-paneled door, her face filled with hurt and fear.

"Tiffany, what happened?" I asked, opening the door.

"I don't know, Kate," she said through tears and confusion. "I don't know. He was fine. We were playing X-box and then he looked at me strangely and said he knew I was cheating on him. He got so mad, so fast. I don't know what happened. I don't know what made him think it or say it. It doesn't make sense." Again, Michael's explosive behavior had come from nowhere.

Mark and I calmed Tiffany as best we could, and when she was less rattled, we asked her to go home. Then we went into Michael's room to talk to him. He was irrational, pacing around his room, shouting at a rapid rate, punching at the furniture and doors, spitting on the walls, and crying through his words.

"Tiffany cheated on me. You guys are against me. I don't have anybody. Nobody understands. You're all out to get me. You want to send me away."

Then he sat down on his bed, shaking his head and rubbing his eyes. When he looked up, he'd stopped crying, and calming said, "I'm not safe here any more. I have to leave. I have to go. I have to go now."

Then he calmed down for a few minutes and we thought that perhaps the storm had passed. It had not.

As quickly as Michael's initial agitation abated, it returned with greater ferocity. He screamed at us, "I know all of you hate me. Well guess what, I hate you too." He punched the walls of his bedroom and the hallway, leaving bloody holes where his battered hands broke through the plaster.

Mark, Monica, and I tried to soothe him with words. "Michael that's not true. We all love you. We always have and we always will. We need to get you some help. We want you to feel better, to be well." He seemed not to hear us.

As Mark and I moved toward him, hoping to touch him, to comfort him, he spat at us. I knew it was an act of aggression just a notch below throwing punches, and felt disgusted, then horrified, by his transformation. Then, before our eyes, he crossed into a realm he'd never before entered. He became homicidal.

Brandishing a knife he'd taken from the kitchen, he threatened to kill Mark, Monica, and me. He quoted dialogue from the movie *The Godfather* and lyrics by Tupac Shakur. He taunted us to come closer so he could cut us. He dared Mark to hit him, "Come on Big Man, hit me. Hit me. What? You too big a pussy to hit me? Such a big man, C'mon, just hit me."

Our Michael was gone. An entirely different person had taken his place. His agitation increased despite our best efforts to calm him. I called Dr. David who said, "This is full-blown mania. He needs to be in the hospital. Call the sheriff if you think you need help and don't take any chances. This is not a safe situation."

Through it all, the four of us shed tears, but Mark, Monica, and I remained eerily calm. Mark left the room for just a few moments to call the hospital for advice on handling the situation. They instructed him to call the sheriff for assistance in getting Michael to the hospital. He did. As this unfolded, I wrote a list of his medications and the names and phone numbers of his doctors and therapist, and then called the hospital to let them know he'd soon be on his way. All the while, Michael pounded walls, cried aloud, and shouted, "Nobody understands. I can't do this any more. I can't stay here. I've got to get out of here."

Naively, I thought an ambulance would arrive and take Michael directly to the hospital. Once again, I was wrong.

When Michael realized the sheriff was en route, he changed tactics. He slammed his door and locked it, and called his friend Joel on the phone. I could hear his end of the conversation and realized he was trying to arrange for a ride away from the house. It was clear that Joel was not cooperating when Michael yelled obscenities into the receiver and slammed down the phone. A few minutes later, he came out of his room dressed in black from head to toe, including a beanie and gloves.

He shouted, "I'm outta here, and I'm ready for the cops," and fled out the back door into the wilderness behind our house.

Shortly after Michael ran off, Joel and another friend, Ray, arrived. Joel looked frightened, "I knew something was really wrong and thought maybe we could help calm Michael down."

"He's run out into the desert, Joel," I told them. "I don't want you to go looking for him. You might not be safe if you find him. He threatened us with a knife. He's not at all himself."

Just then, several Sheriff's Department vehicles pulled up and the officers stormed forward. Mistaking Joel or Ray for Michael, they pulled their guns and ordered them to lie on their stomachs on the driveway. They stayed there for what seemed like an eternity, while Mark and I explained the situation and the officers prepared to search for Michael.

Since he was violent, the sheriff called for back up, K-9 units, and a helicopter to aid in the search of the dense foliage behind our house. I felt like a moviegoer at a screening of a war film.

Uniformed men with radios and weapons moved in and around my home as they took independent statements from Joel, Ray, Monica, Mark, and me. They photographed and documented the bloody holes his fists had left in the walls, the sputum in his room and the hallway, and the knife he'd broken when he slammed it into his closet door. Then they told us to stay in the house, lock all the doors, and under no circumstances to let Michael in.

Only a few minutes later Michael returned with police dogs at his heels. Frightened and worried about the brother she loved so much, Monica couldn't refuse him. She unlocked the door. He came into the kitchen, ranting.

"You motherfuckers. You turned me in to the cops. My own parents turned me in to the cops. Yeah, that's love. You really love me. You called the cops to come take me away." He sobbed and cried out, repeatedly, "My own parents turned me in. You don't love me. You don't love me." Then his demeanor changed. "Well I'm ready for 'em. They don't know who they're messing with." He pulled off his beanie, ran to the side door, and threatened, "I'm gonna take 'em all out."

He opened the door, and ran screaming toward the driveway where several officers stood. He moved forward, yelling obscenities and swinging the knife, "Come and get me mother-fuckers. I dare you, big men. Come on. Come take out the kid."

Then I saw a flash from behind. Michael went down.

For a moment, I thought my son had been shot, but quickly realized he had been hit with a taser. He lay on his stomach, face in the ground, twitching from the electrical current coursing through his body. Because his chemistry was so unbalanced, he, amazingly, rose from the ground and was nearly up before they hit him with another jolt. This time he stayed down. Several officers descended upon him, forcing a knee into the small of his back, handcuffing his wrists together behind his back, and restraining his neck and legs. Then they began to read him his rights and arrest him.

Mark and I jumped into action. We insisted that we'd called them for help in transporting our officially diagnosed mentally ill son to the psychiatric hospital and that they had no right to arrest or charge him with anything. They insisted that laws had been broken and that he had to be charged with domestic violence, physical assault, assault with a deadly weapon, and assaulting a peace officer.

I lost my cool. "If you do not transport our son to the hospital right now, I'll call my lawyer first, your superiors next, and then every newspaper and news station in town. I'll sue every one of you for every penny you've got. You won't work another day in law enforcement when I'm done with you."

Mark stepped in, with an only slightly calmer attitude, "We called the doctor. We called the hospital. We called your Sheriff's substation. We did exactly what each person told us to do. You need to do what we were told you would do."

They began to listen.

I handed the lead officer the list I'd written and suggested he call the doctor and hospital to verify our story. He did.

We stood on the cold January driveway for another forty-five minutes, Michael still on the ground with four officers atop him, while the lead investigator called Michael's doctor, the hospital, and then his commanding officer. Then we waited for that officer to arrive on the scene. As soon as he heard the details of the situation, he instructed his men to take Michael to the emergency room so that the taser probes could be removed and he could undergo a psychiatric evaluation. He also ordered two of the officers to post themselves outside Michael's hospital door until further notice.

They put him in the ambulance, and Mark, Monica, and I followed in our car. The worst was finally over. At the hospital, doctors stabilized and sedated Michael, removed the taser probes, and cleaned and treated his cuts and abrasions. A few hours later, he was transferred to the psychiatric hospital and the police officers were dismissed. He stayed there for a week to further stabilize and begin new medications. Mark and I had to determine the best next step.

During that week, I spent hours every day on the telephone with the people who had thus far participated in his care. I spoke several times a day with our insurance company's case manager as we worked together to identify and select the best inpatient facility for Michael. I called all of the recommended treatment centers within a reasonable distance.

I interviewed intake counselors and shared Michael's medical history. Many refused to consider him as a patient since his eighteenth birthday was only a couple months away. Others suggested I wait until he was eighteen and place him in a longer-duration adult program. We finally found what seemed like the right location only two hours from home, and arranged for his admission.

Michael remained hospitalized for nearly eight weeks while specialists observed, examined, and treated him. Mark and I were allowed to see him twice a week, and the girls could go up for one of those visits. Every time we saw him, our son looked more like his old self. The physical improvements were profound. He gained a little weight, his color improved, and the shine returned to his eyes. I felt hopeful that we were getting him back.

That horrible, traumatic, etched-in-our-memories evening was the beginning of Michael's return to health. Although it served as a beginning, that ordeal could easily have been the end. During a follow-up interview, one of the reporting officers told me we were lucky that a taser-equipped unit had been available that night. If such had not been the case, deadly force would have been used. Michael would have been shot. It took an event of that magnitude for us to appreciate the severity of his problems.

35

Early 2003

"I know of no man of genius who had not to pay, in some affliction or defect either physical or spiritual, for what the gods had given him."
— Max Beerbohm

During his hospital stay, Michael was unable to use substances other than those the doctor prescribed. After a few days, his doctors better understood his body chemistry and reactions with the variable of illicit substances removed. Round-the-clock nursing staff observed and documented his behavior and reactions to medication changes.

He was clearly insomniac, anxious, and depressed. Every third day his care management team met to discuss his progress, reevaluate his treatment plan, and make changes in response to his symptoms. He was a human science experiment, observed, analyzed, and documented. Mark and I received frequent reports and the staff called every time they made a medication change. In just a couple of weeks, Michael improved dramatically.

As part of the comprehensive treatment program, Michael's doctors ordered a brain scan, an EEG, and blood work. As suspected, Michael had a thyroid imbalance and hypoglycemia. It was during this work-up that Michael told of seizures he'd suffered over the previous twelve months. Their cause was never determined, but his doctor suspected head trauma from a series of car accidents, as well as excessive marijuana-use. We learned about the brain damage and the time needed to heal. One doctor warned us that it would take at least a year for everything to settle down, and for Michael's body to repair what it could.

As his health improved, Michael was homesick and sad to be away from friends and family. Nevertheless, he never argued that this was not what he needed or where he needed to be. Now free of illicit substances and beginning to stabilize on his medications, he admitted he'd been racing headlong toward death's door, and that this hospitalization had rerouted him, saving his life. He would never have stopped drinking and drugging in order to separate their effects from his illness. Now, without substances to alter his perceptions, he felt well enough to believe that successful treatment of Bipolar Disorder was possible, and realized that he was not ready to die.

Beginning to recapture his old insights, Michael shared a revelation that his purpose in this world must be unique and important, because, "No matter how hard I tried, I couldn't kill myself, I couldn't make myself die."

When we visited him, first with a therapist and then just as a family, he opened up more than he had in a couple of years. Mark and I learned of several incidents and accidents during in which his life had been in peril. His personal experiences were vast and varied compared to other teens. He knew far more than most others his age.

We heard about a fraternity party where Michael witnessed the shooting of a young college student, and of the rollover accident in which he was a passenger and the father of the driver took his own son to the hospital and sent Michael home with another kid. We learned that he had experimented with nearly every recreational drug available, and that he did so to escape the way he felt, or in hopes that he would die.

We were horrified to learn how much alcohol he'd been drinking, an admission we confirmed when a walk through the land behind our house turned up over a dozen large gin and vodka bottles, exactly where he said they'd be. He consumed one, delivered by friends who wanted to please him, every night he'd been in the new house.

More significantly, we learned about the voices Michael heard at night and how long he'd heard them. We learned that he'd known for a very long time that he, too, had Bipolar Disorder, and that watching Chloe's struggle convinced him that it was a hopeless diagnosis. In addition, we learned how much he loved us, regretted disappointing us, and wanted to make it up to us. He learned how much we loved him, too.

This was a watershed time. Michael was in the hospital, finally receiving the treatment he desperately needed. He took college correspondence courses to complete his high school requirements and participated in several counseling sessions a day.

Encouraged by her relative stability, Chloe, now nearly twenty-one, re-enrolled at the university and began again as a part-time student. Mark and I felt indescribable relief, and my calendar pages were pleasantly void of phone lists and appointments. We traveled to see Michael, went to Monica's soccer games and track meets, visited with Chloe a couple times a week, and settled into the new house.

At the end of February 2003, Michael came home. He saw his therapist once or twice a week, met with Dr. David for medication management, volunteered at a local middle school to fulfill his community service obligation, and quickly finished the independent study classes he'd begun while in the hospital. When he turned eighteen at the end of March, his probation ended, as did mandatory drug testing and required therapy. He was now old enough, and healthy enough, to make his own medical decisions. He continued to take his medications and see his therapist and Dr. David.

Once, a few weeks after Michael returned home from his long hospitalization, his behavior caused great concern. He, Monica, and I were at home one evening. Mark was out of town. Monica and I stood chatting in the kitchen when Michael walked in, taking a handful of paperclips from a drawer.

"What are you doing with all those paperclips?" I asked.

"I'm making a machine."

Finding this a little bizarre, I continued the conversation. "What kind of machine are you making, Michael?"

"I'm making a machine to help the African Americans. The white man has repressed African Americans for years and years, and I've been asked to advocate for them. So, I'm making a machine that will help me do that."

He walked to the kitchen island and set down some of the paperclips while continuing to bend and manipulate the others. Then he spent the next fifteen to twenty minutes giving what seemed like a college lecture on the plight of African Americans in the United States. At some point during this diatribe, he raised his arms, turned his body, and used the word "we."

I asked him, "Michael, are other people here with you?"

"Yeah, they're right here behind me. They're helping me to help the African Americans."

"They're in the kitchen right now?" I asked.

"Yeah, can't you see them?" Then he looked around, mumbled something unintelligible, and returned to his room for the night. The next day he remembered none of it. When I talked to Dr. David, she couldn't explain it, except to say that the episode was obviously laced with grandiosity and that he was clearly psychotic. Nothing like that has ever happened again.

In May 2003, Michael and Chloe took finals and earned exceptional grades. Monica did just as well a week or two later, and looked forward to a summer filled with club soccer and high school volleyball. We celebrated another hallmark with Chloe. She got through the month of May without a hospitalization for the first time since her diagnosis. Her success offered concrete verification that she was better medicated and learning the skills necessary to live well in this world. She was proud of herself and we delighted in her wellness.

Our family returned to weekly pool volleyball games that the last year's turmoil forced us to miss. We spent a week at Newport Beach in June with no crises, and attended Michael's graduation ceremony a week later. Chloe spent the summer working part-time, a thrill after being unable to work for such a long time. Michael worked on the house, completing jobs not yet done since we'd moved in months before. He also enrolled and registered for college courses to begin in August, visiting a few schools before deciding where he wanted to be.

My journal no longer held paragraphs of fear and frustration. I wrote about my interests, my activities, my writing, and my blessings. I still jotted notes about my children and their activities, but they were not plagued by dramatic events or weeks of silence because pain or turmoil prevented my writing. Life developed a rhythm and cadence that nurtured us, and we nurtured each other during the next few precious months.

Most profound during these months was our continued healing. As a family and as individuals, we had suffered a lot of trauma. Now, finally, we entered a period of genuine recovery. We spent time playing cards, going for walks, eating leisurely meals together, and reconnecting with one another. As we regained mutual trust, we let go of past hurts. Some of them we talked about, a lot was simply understood.

We looked at each other with clearer vision and recognized traits and characteristics that made each of us special to the others. We took on few obligations and made minimal plans, choosing to enjoy the moment and appreciate each day. We learned to like one another again, and continued to be grateful for the love that was always there. We had made it through the tough stuff and survived to tell the tale.

36

March 2003

"Learning how to appreciate both pleasant and even seemingly unpleasant experiences is a key to increased fulfillment."
— Mother Theresa

Not long after Michael got out of the hospital, I watched through our family room window as a metalworker, who did several jobs on our new house, spent a few minutes chatting with him. I took Michael to school, and then returned home. When I went out to see how the work was going, this kind man turned off his welder and asked if he could sit in the shade and talk to me for a few minutes. Having seen Michael occasionally during the preceding twelve months, he seemed to understand what we were going through.

"I hope you don't think me too bold, but I need to share my thoughts with you. I want you to know how glad I am that you continued to love and support Michael even though he continued to defy you and disrespect himself. My family is rife with addiction and mental illness and I know how hard it is to keep working toward a solution with someone who doesn't even think there's a problem. It's a lot easier to give up and tell them to get out. I've seen that happen too many times.

"Every Saturday my wife makes sandwiches and I take my boys downtown and we feed the homeless. I try to spend time with the youth, and I'm always saddened and surprised by how many there are. Nearly all of them tell a similar story. They went through the same distress your family has gone through and their parents were either unwilling or unable to continue to care for them. Some of them were beaten and abused, and fled the violence. Some were stubborn, refused to live by the rules, and left. Others just drifted away and no one tried to reel them back in. No matter how it happened, they're on the street, where their addictions grow, their health deteriorates, and they feel alone and unloved.

"As hard as it's been for you, I have no doubt that you saved your son's life. I know people see the surface of things and judge harshly, and you and Mark have probably gotten more than your share of that. I want you to know that people recognize and value what you've done. I'm glad you continued to love and support Michael, and when some time has passed, he'll be glad too."

Grateful, I thanked him, went back into the house, and wept. I wept for what we'd lost, as well as what we'd gained. I wept with joy for what we had, and with gratitude that we'd learned to appreciate it.

37
Late 2003

"Adversity has the effect of eliciting talents, which in prosperous circumstances would have lain dormant."
— Horace

In August 2003, all three of my children returned to school full time. Monica started at the high school campus that Chloe and Michael had attended before her. Michael took his classes at the community college and planned to transfer to the university in the spring. Chloe enrolled full time again, quitting her job so she could focus all her attention on staying healthy and doing well in school. They each had new challenges to face, new difficulties to conquer, and they did so with grace and courage. Dr. David continued to treat both Chloe and Michael. Chloe had craniosacral therapy every week and saw Maria occasionally. Michael maintained a fair sense of balance without seeing a therapist.

Michael still felt a great deal of anxiety at the end of each day, but instead of waiting for Mark and me to go to bed so he could drink a bottle of gin or vodka, he'd ask me to rub his shoulders and head with a massage oil that seemed to calm him. He began sleeping with a soothing sound machine to reduce fear and tension in the night. He also had a boxing bag in the garage to pummel when negative feelings and sensations overwhelmed him. Like Chloe, he learned methods and skills to manage his illness in order to live the life he chose.

I don't want to give the impression that my children will go on to live perfect lives, free of troubles or demands. Chloe is very careful, and forever must be, to take her medications and call her doctor at the first signs of decline. She's not well enough to attend the university every semester, but a degree continues to be her goal. She's had several brief episodes that forced her back home for a few days, where she rested, felt safe, and got herself back to a more stable state. Then she returned to her place and her routine, tackling daily problems like anybody else. It's possible that she'll always need that level of support form us. She knows, as do we, that her health will always be fragile and that she must plan her routine, her schedule, her career, and her life, around the requirements of her health.

Michael has suffered many of the typical, irritating side effects attributed to psychotropic drugs. Initially, he gained weight, continued to have sleep issues, and never felt quite like he ought to. He didn't like Dr. David, so avoided seeing her. After a time it became clear that his struggle to remain stable was too great, and I suggested he switch doctors so that he'd be willing to go. He agreed, and after a thorough search, we found another psychiatrist who was willing to take him as a patient.

During this search, the number of doctors who refused psychiatric patients with a history of substance abuse amazed me. Whom did they think people with drug or alcohol problems, past or current, could see for ongoing healthcare? How did they expect patients like Michael, who worked hard to remain healthy, to do so without medical support? Repeatedly, the inadequacy of medical care for people with mental illness was reinforced.

Seeing a doctor of his own choosing, Michael took control of his health care. He made appointments when necessary and managed his medication. He and his doctor worked together to wean him off all of his meds when he moved into student housing at the university. For several months, he was able to maintain stability, but ultimately went back to the doctor to discuss and then implement new medications.

Rather than feeling hopeless and resorting to illicit or illegal means of alleviating symptoms, he managed his medical care, making choices toward improving rather than masking or detracting his quality of life. He played pick-up soccer and basketball games to ease tension and ate foods that made him feel healthier. He came home for a good night's sleep when nagged by insomnia, and tried to pinpoint activities or foods that made him wakeful. He consciously worked at feeling well.

As time went by, Chloe and Michael both adapted to their routines, and acquired skills and techniques that enable them to live well in spite of chronic mental illness. They have achieved personal milestones, just like those we had proudly annotated in their baby books when they learned to walk, talk, or read. They continued to take big steps on the road to recovery, along life's complicated, interesting, ever-winding path.

Thanksgiving 2003 was a wondrous holiday for our family. We enjoyed a traditional meal together on a beautiful, balmy day. As we sat down to enjoy our celebratory feast, we observed the time-honored tradition of sharing with the rest of the family that for which each was most grateful. Every year this practice made us laugh and sometimes made us cry, but this year was like none before. All three of the children had grown in the realization that life is precious and the love of a family, dear.

We began with Monica: "I'm thankful for my family, and that Michael is feeling good again, and that Chloe is so well."

Then Michael, "Mom and Dad, I'm so glad you're my parents. I don't know any other people who would've been as patient and loving as you've been, putting up with all my crap for such a long time. You're the best parents I know. Thank you for everything you did. I love you."

"I'm glad that Michael and I are both able to be in school, and be in the same room together again without wanting to kill each other," shared Chloe.

We all laughed, appreciating the truth in her words. Mark and I shared our gratitude for new beginnings and our love of each other and our family, and then we tucked in and enjoyed a wonderful meal.

Each of us was keenly aware of what could have been lost since we last went round the table, and each was willing to tell the others of their value, and their love. After agonizing for so long over so many issues, we reveled in the knowledge that we'd all done our best, with what we knew at any given time, and our relationships had not only remained intact, but had flourished.

Two thousand three ended on just as high a note. We'd learned respect for one another, and appreciated each person's uniqueness. Like any siblings, Chloe, Michael, and Monica continued to work out issues of rivalry and differences of opinion, but they were more patient when one or the other wasn't feeling up to par. Monica, especially, developed a very keen sense of how her brother and sister were feeling, and would ask questions out of concern. "Is Chloe getting manic again?" "Is Michael feeling more depressed?" "Is Chloe rapid-cycling?" She tried to learn as much as she could about their illnesses.

Chloe and Michael both became comfortable managing their own wellness and asking for guidance when they needed it. They continued to make doctor's appointments and take their medications, independent of me. Without drugs and alcohol clouding the picture, Michael's illness seemed less severe than Chloe's, and he maintained stability more easily. Nevertheless, they each had to be aware of subtle changes in how they felt in order to head off a crisis.

We had a magical holiday season without the specter of substance abuse or mental instability. This was the first Christmas in many that we had total joy in our world.

Everybody went back to school full time when the 2004 spring semester began, and with only a few days peppered with depression or mania, Chloe and Michael remained healthy and pursued his or her goals. They developed greater insights about dating and socializing, making changes in their routines when they realized their health demanded them. They explored career choices that would suit their gifts and talents as well as their needs. Each of them was able to take a weeklong trip with friends without health issues.

Spring eased into summer, and both Chloe and Michael experienced new and discouraging symptoms. Michael's anxiety and paranoia returned to an unusual extent, robbing him of much-needed sleep and straining relationships with friends. He examined his own actions and began to adjust his behaviors to improve his health. He'd been drinking and smoking pot again, though not to the degree he used to. When his health declined, he partied less, tried to avoid too many late nights, and observed and analyzed his moods and thought processes. Moreover, a big sign of increasing wellness, he was open to Mark's and my observations and assessments of his behaviors and attitudes. He realized we sought not to control, but to support. He grew exceedingly insightful and mature.

Chloe's illness continued to be unstable. While she learned lots of coping techniques, as well as new strategies and skills, medications remained effective for only a few months, and then her doctor had to make adjustments. Anxiety and depression mixed and caused such inner turmoil that she could not cope. Unable to focus or retain information, she again took a medical leave from the university. As before, she felt inadequate and became more depressed. Struggling, she worked hard to consciously control her symptoms and maintain some degree of health. She sought new treatment from a different doctor, hoping that a new perspective might shed new light, and she began taking a different drug combination. She continued to see Maria weekly.

Like many people diagnosed with Bipolar Disorder, in her effort to control symptoms, to feel some control in her life, Chloe began to develop obsessive-compulsive tendencies. She was uncomfortable if her outfits were not perfectly matched. Items on tables had to be aligned at right angles. She (who never before cared if her bed was made) felt terribly anxious if her comforter and pillows were not properly situated. She made detailed lists each day and regimented her activities based upon the lists. She also developed strange eating habits and rapidly lost a large amount of weight.

Maria came to the rescue. She recognized signs of obsessive and compulsive tendencies during one of their weekly meetings. As the one constant in Chloe's medical care, she often held the key to unlocking puzzles created by Chloe's illness. She and Chloe called the new psychiatrist and shared their observations. Together, the three of them decided on a medication change to address the underlying causes of the new symptoms. Working with her medical team, Chloe took control and moved forward, despite setbacks and challenges. Most importantly, she kept herself well enough to avoid suicidal ideations and hospitalization.

Both Chloe and Michael learned that monitoring their illness would forever be necessary. They've continued to grow wiser and stronger, learning to adapt their outer situations to their inner circumstances. Isn't this what each of us does as we learn to get along in this world?

38

One Year Later

"One man scorned and covered with scars
Still strove with his last ounce of courage
To reach the unreachable stars;
And the world was better for this."
    —Don Quixote

A few years ago, when we first learned that Chloe had Bipolar Disorder, Mark and I felt great fear about her prospects in this world. We'd watched his mom suffer for years, misdiagnosed, poorly treated, and usually overmedicated. She became ill long before the medical community knew how to treat mental illness, and spent decades in psychiatric care where she fell victim to well-intentioned, but damaging treatment. She endured electro-shock therapy at dangerously high voltages, and took massive doses of mind and mood-altering drugs.

Her mind permanently transformed. When well, Elizabeth spent her days moving slowly through a routine that included little more than three meals a day, church a couple times a week, occasional fishing trips, and card games. Despite the fact that she often spent time with a group of friends, very little intimate or social contact occurred. Conversations developed around her. People rarely engaged her. She slept twelve to fourteen hours a day, and seemed to exist, but not joyfully live.

When she was particularly unwell, Elizabeth would go to the curb, awaiting a ride that would never come to take her away because someone was trying to hurt her. She sometimes refused to eat because she thought she was being poisoned, leaving Mark's Dad frustrated and helpless as her caretaker. She heard voices, saw things that weren't there, and trusted absolutely no one. She was frightened. She was angry. She was lost. Then she'd spend some time in the hospital and come home with a different mix of medications, and the cycles would start all over again. This was our point of reference when Chloe first got sick.

Fortunately, we learned rather quickly that medicine, even if imperfectly, has evolved. We learned that more effective medications had become available since Mom was treated years ago. It's unfortunate that she didn't benefit from them. However, who am I to judge her path or the value therein? Maybe she, and those of us who loved her, learned important eternal lessons during the time she lived with illness. There is always something to learn.

When I think about this, I also wonder about society's attitudes, my attitudes, regarding differences and disabilities. In an effort to keep our children well, Mark and I researched and investigated every means of controlling, even eradicating Bipolar Disorder. Millions of parents have done the same for hundreds of other diseases and disorders. We want our loved ones free from suffering and hardship. We want the illnesses, the disabilities, gone. I now know, without a doubt, that this cut-and-dry approach is morally, ethically, and spiritually wrong. In our efforts to love and support, we have to be aware of, and careful about, the messages we send and the goals we seek.

If we believe that disabilities must be altered or abolished, then we imply that the absence of disability equals a good life. But does it? Because if that's true, one might deduce that anyone with a disability is inferior. That line of reasoning leads to a horrible, deeply disturbing, and dangerous arena. I hate to imagine a human race that no longer gives rise to brilliant individuals like Irving Berlin, Michelangelo, Sylvia Plath, Mark Rothko, Vincent Van Gogh, Tennessee Williams, Walt Whitman, and Virginia Wolf, all of whom likely had Bipolar Disorder.

Think of the other great minds whose varied illnesses and disabilities were fundamental in developing the people they became and the contributions they made. We cannot disregard the fact that challenges mold us and make us better. We cannot aim to rid the human race of these differences. I would fight even harder against that medical and ethical direction than I have fought to keep my children alive and well. Disability does not require solution or abolition, but understanding, and when necessary, temperance to allow the disabled to function more fully.

In the end, I've learned that acceptance is the key. I want my children to be well enough to find joy in their lives. I don't seek a cure, but a moderation of symptoms that allows them to live happily. I want them to interact with a peer group of their choice, contribute to the world through their gifts and talents, and develop and enjoy supportive and fulfilling relationships. I want them to feel the kind of connection to another human being that Mark and I share.

In addition to strengthening our commitment to one another, this journey through madness has taught Mark and me to embrace differences and revel in the beauty they create. It has taught us to love more deeply and freely than we thought possible. It has shined a bright and brilliant light on what is most precious.

We know that our children will cycle and experience difficult times. We know that Michael must forever work hard to maintain a healthy relationship with medications, drugs, and alcohol. Chloe must vigilantly assess her lifestyle and choices in order to remain balanced and functional.

Bipolar Disorder is a chronic mental illness. It does not go away. Chloe and Michael will always have it. It will forever alter their lives, and as a result, will alter ours too. Nevertheless, we embrace the experience and anticipate future legs of the journey because we know that this world, this life, offers everybody opportunities to learn and grow and evolve.

Each one of us will live through life-altering experiences, and if wisdom prevails, we learn from them. We make the best of it. We improve ourselves and help others to do the same. We leave judgment and anger behind, and move into a place of loving acceptance and advocacy where our actions enrich and improve the lives of others living in similar circumstance. We learn as much as we can and then share what we've learned.

Hoping to contribute to that leaning, and help move medical and technical knowledge forward, both Chloe and Michael agreed to participate in a genetic study conducted by the Juvenile Bipolar Research Foundation. Their DNA, along with the DNA of several hundred other siblings with their diagnosis, is being studied in an effort to find the particular chromosomes responsible for the illness. After mailing their DNA saliva kits back to the Foundation, we had a lengthy conversation about the possible results and outcomes. What if Bipolar Disorder could be eradicated? What if they could undergo gene therapy and rid themselves of the illness?

Interestingly, neither of my children would choose that course. They would not change what they now see as an elemental part of who they are. At this point, despite the obvious difficulties, they consider Bipolar Disorder a factor in the genetic mix that makes them unique individuals. One of them, however, would consider using technology to prevent the illness's emergence in future children. The other thinks it's wrong to manipulate fate. Both agree that research and medical advances are vital so that every person affected by Bipolar Disorder has the opportunity to make those very personal decisions for him or herself. They agree that research will lead to better medications and treatments, and offer continued hope.

Every month that passes brings new hope for the mentally ill. Every time researchers test new medication on a population of non-responding patients, new possibilities for wellness emerge. Hope abounds if you only have faith. Without hesitation, I encourage my children to hang on through the hard times since a miracle treatment might be in the works.

Lately, we've investigated orthomolecular treatments for both mental illness and addiction. Simplified, the goal of orthomolecular medicine is to restore the natural, health-maintaining chemical balance of the brain and body through supplements and nutrition rather than medication. Actress/activist Margot Kidder first suggested this treatment approach to me, and credits it with her ten-plus years of wellness after decades of mania and depression. Among others, Dr. Joan Matthews Larson, founder of Health Recovery Center in Minneapolis, has created treatment protocols based on orthomolecular medicine that offer promising results. The field seems to be growing.

The children continue to work toward their goals. Chloe takes a few classes at the university every semester and hopes to move into the workforce, using her skills as an artist, editor, or

magazine designer. These fields would allow the flexibility
demanded by her illness and concomitant symptoms. She no
longer fears the future as she used to. She is gradually gaining
confidence.

Michael has a few more semesters at the university and
dreams of working in Mexico. He speaks Spanish fluently,
admires many of the Mexican values and lifestyle, and plans a
career in which he can fuse his skills and charisma to improve
business relations between Mexicans and Americans.

And Monica is well. Because we know she could still
become ill, Mark and I watch and listen carefully for the telltale
signs of emerging Bipolar Disorder. We take comfort in the
knowledge that both Chloe and Michael exhibited severe signs
and symptoms by her age. They both knew something was
terribly wrong long before the rest of us figured it out and right
now, Monica has no symptoms. Yes, it could still happen. If it
does, we're better prepared. We know our way around the
mental health care system. We know good doctors, and we
know a lot about medicines and side effects. Mostly, we know
we can do it. For now, she is well. We are well. And the future
seems sweet.

Remember the truth in the fortune cookie:
"Those who do not taste the bitter never taste the sweet."
Savor life.

APPENDIX I-a
SYMPTOMS OF BIPOLAR DISORDER
MANIA*

— Overly happy or euphoric mood
— Heightened senses, especially hearing and smell
— Pressed speech — talking faster, louder, or beginning new thoughts before finishing
— Racing thoughts
— Distractibility
— Irritability
— Quickly shifting moods
— Decreased inhibitions
— Increased sense of importance
— Grandiosity
— Paranoia, paranoid delusions
— Unrealistic fear or lack of fear, risk-taking
— Increased physical activity
— Decreased need for sleep
— Spending sprees or foolish investments
— Increased sexual activity
— Increased drug and/or alcohol use
— Increased drive to write or create

*Adapted from *Bipolar Disorders: A Guide to Helping Children and Adolescents* by Mitzi Waltz, O'Reilly & Associates, Inc., Sebastopol, CA, 2000.

APPENDIX I-b
SYMPTOMS OF BIPOLAR DISORDER
DEPRESSION *

- Deep sadness
- Loneliness regardless of social setting, situation
- Hopelessness
- Physical aches and pains
- Significant weight change
- Inability to experience pleasure
- Slow or impaired thought processes
- Inability to concentrate
- Memory and recall difficulties
- Preoccupation with death and dying
- Thoughts or visions of suicide (suicidal ideation)
- Decreased self esteem
- Feelings of worthlessness, failure, excessive guilt, self-hatred
- Reduction in physical activity
- Sleep disturbances
- Physical exhaustion

*Adapted from *Bipolar Disorders: A Guide to Helping Children and Adolescents* by Mitzi Waltz, O'Reilly & Associates, Inc., Sebastopol, CA, 2000.

APPENDIX I-c
SYMPTOMS OF BIPOLAR DISORDER
MIXED STATES*

— Any combination of symptoms from either category, such as depression with anxiety or mania with deep sadness
— Self mutilation, such as cutting, cigarette burns, or hitting head or fists against walls
— Raging
— Aggressive posturing

*Adapted from *Bipolar Disorders: A Guide to Helping Children and Adolescents* by Mitzi Waltz, O'Reilly & Associates, Inc., Sebastopol, CA, 2000.

APPENDIX I-d
SYMPTOMS OF BIPOLAR DISORDER
PSYCHOSIS*

- Bizarre, difficult to explain behavior
- Unusual or unrealistic beliefs
- Auditory hallucinations
- Visual hallucinations
- Difficult to understand speech
- Impulsive, dangerous, or irrational behaviors
- Physical and mental slowness
- Extreme apathy
- Lack of emotional responses, flat affect

*Adapted from *Bipolar Disorders: A Guide to Helping Children and Adolescents* by Mitzi Waltz, O'Reilly & Associates, Inc., Sebastopol, CA, 2000.

APPENDIX II
RECOMMENDED READING

Amador, X., and Johanson, A. (2000). *I Am Not Sick. I Don't Need Help: Helping the Seriously Mentally Ill Accept Treatment. A Practical Guide for Families and Therapists.* New York: Vida Press.

Berren, M. R., Ph.D. (2004). *A Sourcebook for Families Coping With Mental Illness.* shoestopm@yahoo.com.

Campbell, B. M. (2005). *72-Hour Hold.* New York: Alfred K. Knopf.

Earley, P. (2006). *Crazy: A Father's Search Through America's Mental Health Madness.* New York: The Berkley Publishing Group.

Fawcett, J., M.D., Golden, B., Ph.D., and Rosenfeld, N. (2000). *New Hope for People with Bipolar Disorder.* Roseville, CA: Prima Publishing.

Goodwin, F. K., M.D., and Jamison, K. R., Ph.D. (1990, rev. 2006). *Manic-Depressive Illness.* New York: Oxford University Press.

Jamison, K. R. (1995). An *Unquiet Mind, A Memoir of Moods and Madness.* New York: Vintage Books.

Jamison, K. R. (1999). *Night Falls Fast, Understanding Suicide.* New York: Alfred K. Knopf.

Jamison, K. R. (1994). *Touched With Fire, Manic-Depressive Illness and The Artistic Temperament.* New York: Free Press Paperbacks.

Larson, J. M., Ph.D. (1999). *Depression Free, Naturally.* New York: Ballantine Wellspring.

Larson, J. M., Ph.D. (1997). *Seven Weeks to Sobriety.* New York:

Ballantine Wellspring.

Marohn, S. (2003). *The Natural Medicine Guide to Bipolar Disorder.* Charlottesville, VA: Hampton Roads Publishing Company, Inc.

Miklowitz, D. J., Ph.D., and Goldstein, M. J. (1997). *Bipolar Disorder, A Family-Focused Treatment Approach.* New York: The Guilford Press.

Miklowitz, D. J., Ph.D. (2002). *The Bipolar Survival Guide, What You and Your Family Need To Know.* New York: The Guilford Press.

Mondimore, F. M., M.D. (1999). *Bipolar Disorder, A Guide for Patientsand Families.* Baltimore, MD: The Johns Hopkins University Press.

Murphree, R. H., DC, CNS. (2005). *Treating & Beating Anxiety and Depression with Orthomolecular Medicine.* Birmingham, AL: Harrison and Hampton Publishing, Inc.

Oliwenstein, L. (2004). *Taming Bipolar Disorder.* New York: Alpha Books.

Papolos, D. F., M.D. and Papolos, J. (2006). *The Bipolar Child.* Third Edition. NewYork: Broadway Books.

Roger, J., and McBay, M. (2005). *Spiritual High: Alternatives to Drugs and Substance Abuse.* Los Angeles: Mandeville Press.

Torrey, E. F., M.D., and Knable, M. B. (2002). *Surviving Manic Depression, A Manual on Bipolar Disorder for Patients, Families and Providers.* New York: D.O. Basic Books.

Waltz, M. (2002). *Adult Bipolar Disorders, Understanding Your Diagnosis and Getting Help.* Sebastapol, CA: O'Reilly and Associates, Inc.

Waltz, M. (2000). *Bipolar Disorders, A Guide to Helping Children & Adolescents.* Sebastapol, CA: O'Reilly and Associates, Inc.

Whybrow, P. C., M.D. (1997). *A Mood Apart. The Thinker's Guide to Emotion and Its Disorders.* New York: HarperPerrenial.

APPENDIX III
USEFUL RESOURCES

American Association of Child and Adolescent Psychiatry
3615 Wisconsin Avenue, Northwest
Washington DC 20016
(202) 966-7300 / www.aacap.org

American Psychiatric Association
1400 K Street, Northwest
Washington, DC 20005
(888) 357-7924 / www.psych.org

American Psychological Association
750 First Street, Northeast
Washington, DC 20002
(800)374-3120 / www.apa.org

The Bipolar Child Website
www.bipolarchild.com

Center for Improvement of Human Functioning
3100 North Hillside Avenue
Wichita, KS 62719
(316) 682-3100 / www.brightspot.org

Child and Adolescent Bipolar Foundation
www.cabf.org or www.bpkids.org

Depression and Bipolar Support Alliance
730 North Franklin, Suite 501
Chicago, IL 60610-9961
(800) 826-3632 / www.DBSAlliance.org

Depression and Related Affective Disorders Association
The Johns Hopkins Hospital, Meyer 3-181
600 North Wolfe Street
Baltimore, MD 21287
(410) 955-4647 /www.med.jhu.edu/drada

Health Recovery Center
3255 Hennepin Ave. S.
Minneapolis, MN 55408
(800) 554-9155 / www.healthrecovery.com

NAMI (previously National Alliance for the Mentally Ill)
2107 Wilson Boulevard, Suite 300
Arlington, VA 22201-3402
(800) 950-6264 / www.nami.org

National Alliance for Research on Schizophrenia and Affective
Disorders
www.mhsource.com/narsad.html

National Institute of Mental Health
6001 Executive Boulevard
Bethesda, MD 20892
(800) 421-4211 / www.nimh.nih.gov

National Mental Health Association
1201 Prince Street
Alexandria, VA 22314
(800) 969-6642 / www.nmha.org

Pfeiffer Treatment Center
4575 Weaver Parkway
Warrenville, Illinois
(866) 504-6076 / www.hriptc.org

Substance Abuse and Mental Health Services
www.samhsa.gov

APPENDIX V
OTHERS DIAGNOSED WITH BIPOLAR DISORDER

Buzz Aldrin
Hans Christian Anderson
Honore de Balzac
Charles Baudelaire
Ned Beatty
Irving Berlin
William Blake
Napoleon Bonaparte
Robert Burns
Lord Byron
Agatha Christie
Winston Churchill
Samuel Clemens/ Mark Twain
Rosemary Clooney
Kurt Cobain
Francis Ford Coppola
Noel Coward
Isak Denisen
Charles Dickens
Emily Dickenson
Robert Downey Jr.
Patti Duke
T.S. Eliot
Ralph Waldo Emerson
William Faulkner
Carrie Fisher
F. Scott Fitzgerald
Paul Gauguin
Mark Rothko
Anne Sexton
Graham Greene
George Frideric Handel
Ernest Hemingway
Hermann Hesse

Victor Hugo
Henry James
John Keats
Margot Kidder
Otto Klemperer
Charles Lamb
Jack London
Robert Lowell
Gustav Mahler
Kristy McNichol
Herman Melville
Michelango
Edna St. Vincent Millay
Charles Mingus
Edvard Munch
Georgia O'Keefe
Eugene O'Neill
Sylvia Plath
Edgar Allan Poe
Jackson Pollock
Cole Porter
Ezra Pound
Charlie Pride
Sergey Rachmaninoff
Theodore Roethke
Robert Louis Stevenson
Peter Tchaikovsky
Alfred, Lord Tennyson
Dylan Thomas
Leo Tolstoy
Vincent Van Gogh
Tennessee Williams
Walt Whitman
Virginia Woolf